hal a. huggins, d.d.s., m.s.
&
thomas e. levy, m.d., j.d.

UNINFORMED CONSENT

the hidden dangers in dental care

HAMPTON ROADS
PUBLISHING COMPANY, INC.

for the evolving human spirit

Cover design by Marjoram Productions
Cover Painting by Frank Pedrick (Index Stock Photography)

For information write:

Hampton Roads Publishing Company, Inc.
134 Burgess Lane
Charlottesville, VA 22902

Or call: 804-296-2772
FAX: 804-296-5096
e-mail: hrpc@hrpub.com
Web site: http://www.hrpub.com

If you are unable to order this book from your local
bookseller, you may order directly from the publisher.
Quantity discounts for organizations are available.
Call 1-800-766-8009, toll-free.

Library of Congress Catalog Card Number: 98-71590

ISBN 1-57174-117-8

10 9 8 7 6 5 4 3 2 1

Printed on acid-free recycled paper in Canada

TABLE OF CONTENTS

Part IV Post Dental Revision: The Recovery Process is Only Beginning

Consent

Foreword by James L. Merrill

Freedom of choice is a cornerstone of democracy. That each individual should decide the course of his or her own life is an ideal most people cherish. Making good choices requires more than freedom, however. A meaningful choice also requires individual knowledge and access to information. People cannot make wise decisions without being aware of the alternatives available to them and without knowing the consequences of their options. American law recognizes and supports this philosophy through the doctrine of informed consent.

In a typical medical context, informed consent requires a doctor to obtain a patient's permission prior to a treatment or an operation. For the patient's permission to be valid, the patient must be aware of the nature of his or her ailment, the proposed treatment, the available alternatives to the proposed treatment, and any "substantial risks" involved in undergoing the proposed treatment and each alternative. A "substantial risk" is often defined as one that is significant to a patient in deciding whether or not to submit to a particular treatment.

The law of informed consent varies among states because it is in large part a creature of state, not federal, law. Depending on the state, failure to obtain a patient's consent when required can subject a physician to greater legal liabilities to patients, additional insurance costs, and licensing sanctions. As a result, obtaining informed consent when required is normally standard procedure in medical practice.

While informed consent normally relates to public health, the ideal behind it is not restricted to the practice of medicine. We have over-the-counter medicines, cigarettes, and alcohol with warnings about the potential adverse consequences of their use. Federal law now requires warnings to workers about additional risks in the workplace. The "Community Right to Know" amendment to the Superfund toxic sites cleanup law even requires that the public have access to central inventories of information about the amounts and locations of toxic materials in the community.

This latter requirement is particularly interesting because dentistry typically involves the permanent implantation of materials in a patient's mouth. Many of dentistry's materials are toxic and regulated in the environment as hazardous substances. In a patient's mouth, however, these same materials are hardly regulated at all. Indeed, we have the right to know if mercury and other toxic components of dental amalgam are present in our neighborhoods but not if they are in our mouths. This is because, until recently, informed consent and the practice of dentistry have had little to do with one another.

This situation is changing, however. A growing number of dentists are declining to place mercury amalgam or are advising their patients of the risks and alternatives (and obtaining patient consent) before doing so. In addition, California recently adopted a law bringing dentistry and informed consent closer together.

California's new Senate Bill 934 requires the Board of Dental Examiners to prepare a fact sheet describing the various dental restorative materials available for use. The fact sheet must also contain "a reference to encourage discussion between the patient and dentist regarding materials and to inform the patient of his or her options." The law does not require such a discussion but encourages it. The California Dental Board must make the fact sheet available to all licensed dentists in the state and update the fact sheet as determined necessary by the Board. While California does not require informed consent, it certainly nudges dentistry toward the practice.

California's new disclosure law applies only within its borders, however; other states have not yet considered or adopted this approach. Federal law could also require disclosure for the benefit of people nationwide, but it does not yet do so. Adopting informed consent in dentistry will require hard work and sustained demands by the people for their rights to know more. I hope that this book will stimulate those efforts.

James L. Merrill is a former Environmental Protection Agency attorney and advisor to the Office of Enforcement and Compliance Monitoring. He is currently in private practice in Colorado Springs, Colorado, where his special interests are toxic wastes and environmental law.

Introduction

Many "incurable" diseases may be incurable, but they may also be preventable. This prevention is not by using a multitude of modern "miracle" drugs, but directly by you. There is a price to pay. You must become informed and educated. You must be willing to take responsibility for your own health. Few people in the "establishment" are willing to discuss this situation because of the many legal implications and large sums of insurance money at risk.

What preventable diseases are we addressing?

Although the list is much longer, prominent ones included are multiple sclerosis, lupus, Alzheimer's, Parkinson's, Lou Gehrig's disease, and breast cancer. There are many more symptom clusters lacking formal disease names. These include chronic fatigue, memory problems, emotional instability, "female problems," and indigestion. Kids aren't spared, either. Some of their more preventable afflictions include hyperkinesis, attention deficit, birth defects, lowered grade point average, and visual disturbances.

And how can one avoid these problems? The simple answer is to avoid the cause. Frequently the cause is exposure to one or more toxins from dental materials in the mouth. The situation becomes more complicated when you've already been primarily exposed, and you want to eliminate the current exposure. Such dental toxins include mercury, cadmium, copper, zinc, beryllium, nickel, phenol, and the toxic wastes generated by anaerobic bacteria.

Most dentists are entirely unaware of either the contents of the dental materials they implant *or* the potential consequences of those materials after they get into your body. Manufacturers, trade magazines (such as the *Journal of the American Dental Association*), and editorial opinions continue to reassure dentists that these toxic materials are safe while in the mouth. These dental materials are known to you as silver fillings, crowns or caps, bridges, implants, children's chrome crowns, orthodontic braces, retainers, root canals, and the necessary removal of wisdom teeth.

Can anything be done if you already have some of the symptoms or diseases we have mentioned? That depends. It depends on how severely ill you already are, and on how reactive your immune system is to the materials that you already have in your mouth. It depends on the skills of the practitioners who are treating you, and on how well they understand dental toxicity and the unique problems associated with dental toxicity. It depends on how dedicated *you* are to being an active participant in the treatment process. The information in this book is not about magic bullets or instant cures. It only outlines a road to possible success and invites you to travel that road.

The information in this book may be your first introduction to the concept that your mouth could be a toxic waste site worthy of fines from the Environmental Protection Agency. Don't leave your health in your dentist's hands and assume that all will be fine. Become informed and take an active role in your full and complete consent to all that will be implanted into your mouth. Many of the toxic preparations used in your mouth will be less expensive and more durable than the safer alternatives. But you must decide at the outset which is of the most importance to you: The life of the filling, or the life of the patient (you). The choice is yours alone to make. Good reading and God bless.

Personally Speaking:
The Medical Aspects of Dental Toxicity

Thomas E. Levy, M.D., J.D.

The Meeting

I met Dr. Huggins in July of 1993 at the Extraordinary Science Conference, an annual event sponsored by the International Tesla Society in Colorado Springs. We both had already made presentations at the conference, Dr. Huggins on the toxicity of mercury amalgams, and I on the effects of unipolar magnetic fields on biological systems. My own limited work with such magnetic applications had already made it unequivocally clear to me that mainstream medicine was often more concerned with protecting the status quo than with opening itself to new ideas from outside its ranks. Having already read Dr. Huggins' book *It's All in Your Head,* the concept of mercury toxicity from amalgam fillings was not a completely novel concept to me, and I even felt that much of the book followed logical and straightforward scientific concepts. However, the application of those concepts to the standard practice of adult cardiology seemed minimal at best. Nevertheless, I appreciated the opportunity to meet

15

Dr. Huggins, if only because I felt even then that there were some things that I could learn from him. The International Tesla Society, after all, specializes in bringing forward-thinking scientists from across the world to discuss new and radical ways to create energy and promote nontraditional medical treatments. My mind was open and ready to learn, even if my traditional scientific training was prepared to throw up roadblocks whenever something did not synchronize with all the information that I already "knew" to be true. Scientific arrogance can be tough to shake. Every time I confront a colleague with what I know today, I try to remember my own perspective back on that summer day.

After having an informative discussion with Dr. Huggins during that first meeting, I remember commenting to him that it certainly seemed logical enough that mercury amalgam fillings could harm one's health in a variety of ways, which I had taken to be the primary point in his book. Feeling in perfect health at age 42, I proceeded to ask him whether he felt I should have my amalgams removed. His sarcastic reply at the time was simply: "Only if you want to stay healthy." Although I now know that Dr. Huggins can often resort to sarcasm to make a point, at the time I felt that such a reply was arrogant, at the least. But I never forgot that comment, either.

Several months later, I had the opportunity to tour Dr. Huggins' office. As he seemed to be a sincere and educated person, and the clinical results he reported in his book were so fantastic, it seemed a personal visit was the next logical step of my investigation into the effects of dental toxicity. I can no longer remember if I really had anticipated being as amazed as I was. Especially impressive were many of the before-and-after videotape interviews that were conducted on each patient who went through Dr. Huggins' dental revision program. Some of the most impressive tapes showed neurological patients, many having multiple sclerosis, relearning how to take baby steps for the first time in months or even years. These results would often begin to take place only after a portion of the program was completed. Literally, some wheelchair-bound patients were once again becoming minimally ambulatory, despite their neurologists' pronouncements that such improvements simply cannot occur after such advanced neurological degeneration. Although I would later find out that such amazing improvements were only the tip of the iceberg, my traditional medical knowledge base had suffered a major earthquake to its foundations, and my life, both professionally and personally, would never be the same again.

Hitting Close to Home

Six months after the conference and my initial meeting with Dr. Huggins, my "perfect health" suddenly collapsed. I began to have pounding headaches for the first time in my life, and when my office assistant finally took my blood pressure, the reading was 150/112. Such a reading on a patient in my earlier days of practice would have had me considering immediate hospitalization. As I was the patient, I had no intention of hospitalizing myself, but I was scared. Scared as hell. Treating hypertension, or blood pressure elevation, is the bread and butter of the clinical cardiologist, and I knew all too well that such a diagnosis was a diagnosis for life. You only get "rid" of high blood pressure when you take medicine every day for the rest of your life, sustain a massive heart attack or stroke, go into congestive heart failure, or die. Dietary measures and lifestyle changes might moderate mild high blood pressure, but a bottom number of 112 already represented an advanced condition, and I realized my options were limited. I could start medicating myself promptly, or I could pretend that everything was fine. The third and best option would not become apparent to me for several more months. Very reluctantly, I began to take medication. Gradually, my blood pressure came under only fair control. It seemed my high blood pressure was going to require multiple medications or substantially higher dosing of one medication to reach acceptable control. Depression began to superimpose itself on everything else.

Since I had no idea that my high blood pressure could be resolved short of a medical catastrophe, I became preoccupied with how quickly my "perfect health" had deteriorated to the point of requiring prescription medicine for the rest of my life. I did consider that the high blood pressure had been precipitated by my mercury amalgams, as mercury has been shown to have a direct vaso-constricting, blood pressure-elevating effect in animal studies. I simply did not consider that removing the amalgams could also "remove" the high blood pressure. Instead, I started to fixate on all those before-and-after videos of Dr. Huggins' wheelchair-bound patients. Multiple sclerosis had always scared and intrigued me, especially in its seemingly arbitrary manner of striking down young people who appeared to be in the best of health. To go from health to a wheelchair now no longer seemed just a theoretical possibility for one of my patients. I now felt that anything could happen to me at any time, and I wasn't eager to expose my now increasingly fragile health to one extra day of avoidable toxicity.

The Consult

Soon I found myself sitting in front of Dr. Huggins, undergoing a consultative evaluation. He kept on talking about diet, lifestyle, supplementation, and what seemed to be an endless stream of peripheral issues. But I was plagued with toxicity! Why was I being subjected to all of these marginally relevant topics? I again thought about the patients' videotapes, and even about a few of the conversations that I had had with several excited patients who had partially completed the dental revision program at Dr. Huggins' clinic. I concluded that he at least had the right to present to me whatever he felt important.

Then Dr. Huggins noted my one root canal tooth on X-ray. The tooth had never bothered me, and functionally it seemed to work perfectly.

"That'll have to come out," he commented almost as an aside.

"But it doesn't hurt. It's perfectly fine," I protested. "How can you tell it's bad, anyway? What are you seeing on the X-ray?"

"Toxins don't show up on X-ray," Huggins replied. "I see that it is a root canal, and that's all I really need to know. Some root canals are less toxic than others, but they all do more harm than mercury could ever hope to."

I was reeling. I came in to get some fillings changed, and now I was getting a perfectly good tooth amputated. "It *has* to?" I weakly queried.

"Not much point in even messing with the amalgams if we leave that root canal. But we'll do whatever you want to do."

Again thinking of the results that I knew Dr. Huggins had already achieved, and desiring to just put my trust in someone and not research the facts for myself (*not* a good idea in general), I barely whispered back, "Okay, you're the boss; do what you think is best."

I wasn't remotely prepared for what was to happen next.

The Medicine Mindset

I quickly realized after my dental revision was completed that low-grade, chronic symptomatology tends to be ignored. Unless you are frankly ill, you consider yourself to be well, especially when your chronically compromised state of "normalcy" is shared with you by most of the population. If everybody gets headaches, arthritis, gastritis, and brain fog from time to time, it must be part of the normal aging process that just has to be accepted. Today when I talk to people who are curious about what effect dental toxicity might be having on them, the majority of them consider "good health" to include the effective symptomatic control of one or more chronic illnesses with prescription medicine. High blood pressure, migraines, diabetes, and arthritis are commonly accepted by most people as the penalty to be paid for reaching their forties. If they can take a handful of drugs and feel well, then that will satisfy their notion of being in good health.

Nothing could be further from the truth. If you are on prescription medicines, you are *not* well, even if you are holding most of the symptoms at bay. Dying in your seventies after spending the last twenty to thirty years of your life with one or more chronic diseases may be the pattern shared by the majority of the population, but it is not good health, and you do not have to settle for it.

The Response

I soon realized that the "perfect health" that I had enjoyed prior to the onset of my headaches and high blood pressure left a lot to be desired. Following my dental revision, my general health improved in such an undeniable fashion that it became apparent to me that I had been dealing with significant, not minor, health problems for a long time. My second medical education was just beginning.

Within days of the completion of my dental work, my blood pressure readings were in the normal range. For a few months, the bottom number would periodically stray into the minimally elevated range. After this initial period of adjustment (and detoxification, to be specifically addressed later), my numbers were normal whenever checked, and they have remained so for some five years now. I would later learn, in my subsequent work with Dr. Huggins, that high blood pressure was routinely completely resolved after a successful total dental revision. The vast majority of hypertensive patients normalized off of all medication. The remaining few patients with severely elevated blood pressures, only poorly controlled on multiple, highly dosed medications, would demonstrate excellent control on relatively little medication. Usually they would trade in their many medicines for a relatively low dose of a single medicine. This reversibility of hypertension would have been mind-numbing enough had there been no other accompanying changes in my health. But my astonishment was only beginning.

Although I had never perceived my energy to be low, it now skyrocketed. I had always played tennis or racquetball and routinely worked ten- to twelve-hour days, so chronic fatigue simply could not be one of my problems.

Yet, within a few months following my dental work, I began to notice that I was becomingly increasingly impatient with waiting for the hospital elevator while making rounds. Instead, I would more routinely take the stairs. Further, I would literally bolt up the stairs, taking several steps at a time. Not too long afterward, I remembered that taking the stairs had always made me quickly short of breath and caused my heart to race for several minutes after I had reached my desired floor. No more. Just as you climb a mountain because it's there, I was taking the stairs because I *could*. The elevated altitude of Colorado Springs that had been blamed for my short-windedness for almost three years was completely innocent. Waking up in the morning was no longer a daily torture. I no longer wished the sleep could go on indefinitely and cursed the shattering sound of the alarm. Sleep once again rejuvenated me, and it was as normal to spring from bed as it was to bolt up the hospital stairs.

My surging energy and returning breath were not the only dramatic clinical changes. The ability to think clearly, analyze precisely, and remember completely began to return. This was a real shocker to me, since I was a specialist in both internal medicine and cardiology, and I certainly felt my patients were getting the best of care. It was then I humbly realized that even professions requiring many years of preparation could be practiced with cookbook approaches. Novel, intuitive thinking was not really necessary. I realized that cardiology, along with all the other extensively schooled professions, could be satisfactorily practiced with varying degrees of cognitive impairment, or "brain fog." My improvement in health was closely attended by a decline in intellectual arrogance.

Until a full six months had passed following my dental revision, I did not realize just how much my mind had recovered. Although I had read numerous books during the course of my education, a critical review of my recent years revealed that my reading amounts had become almost inconsequential, limited to brief articles, and rarely ever extending to full books. I was now devouring books that had interested me enough to be purchased, but had nevertheless rested undisturbed on my shelves for many years. Difficulty in concentrating and remembering had almost stopped all significant reading for me, and I hadn't even realized it. Having read roughly ten books in the past five years of my life before my dental work, I now realized that I had since devoured roughly fifty books, most of them highly technical works involving my new passions: toxicology and nutrition. And what was even more gratifying was the rebirth of my ability to remember. Names, dates, journal titles, statistical data—all of this was so much more readily accessible from memory than it had ever been before. A few years later, using a commercially available memory course, I completely memorized all the elements on the periodic table in just a few hours, just to prove to myself that I could do it. My rejuvenated mind also allowed me to complete law school in 1998, an undertaking that would have been completely impossible for me a few short years earlier. My empathy and compassion for my fellow toxic human beings would now often overwhelm me, as I could more clearly perceive the daily struggle that so many people endured, battling against the burden of so many *unconsented* toxins, administered in the name of good health by people who should be trustworthy.

My previously "perfect health" had also been compromised by increasingly severe stomach pain and periodic difficulty swallowing for the prior year or two. A tube down my throat was not too far away, as my tennis buddy was a gastroenterologist, and he was more than willing to check it out for me at any time. I just wasn't sure that "diagnosing" the problem was going to make any real difference in the clinical management, so I continued to hold off. I did recall, however, how my grandmother had suffered greatly with multiple dilations to her lower esophagus.

There had to be something better than just waiting for the seemingly inevitable outcome to occur, even though I had no idea what that could be at the time. However, after my dental revision, this problem promptly and completely disappeared. On learning of this and what I had done, my doctor friend just nervously commented, "That's interesting," and never made another comment about it. As would happen many times in subsequent years, I was getting the opportunity to witness how the old me would have reacted only a few years earlier. More than once, I could remember myself saying, "If it's really good, it'll make its way into the *New England Journal of Medicine,* and all the doctors will know about it."

A few years later, I had my routine eye examination. My astigmatism, which my ophthalmologist had told me was irreversible, had clearly lessened. I told him what I had been through, and once again, I heard that familiar refrain, "That's interesting." I sent him scientific information on the subject, but he never attempted to discuss any of the issues with me. For that matter, I sent detailed information on this whole process to about thirty of my closest friends and colleagues across the country. I have yet to get a call or letter from any of them wanting to discuss the issues, wanting to get more information, or wanting just to comment on how sad it was to see that I had gone crazy.

Was Seeing Really Believing?

In the immediate months following my dental revision, my biggest adjustments were mental and emotional. As each day went by, my assimilation of the previously unrealized mountains of information on heavy metal and dental toxicity steadily progressed. So much of my previous medical training seemed almost irrelevant now, as I was discovering that so many diseases that traditional medicine was incapable of helping or reversing would respond to the removal of dental toxicity. On a rare occasion, a disease process that had always been labeled "incurable" appeared to disappear completely, at least from the perspective of blood chemistries and clinical appearance. Can the incurable sometimes be cured? Who knows? I just know that if someone stops coughing without cough suppressants, then the cough is gone. And when symptoms sometimes disappear, modern medicine considers the disease to be resolved, or at least sent into indefinite remission. More than anything else, my traditional schooling gave me the best possible backdrop to "fill in the blanks," satisfactorily allowing me to resolve so many questions that had long bothered me about the causes of so many different disease processes. What was initially enormously frustrating later dovetailed into a better appreciation of diseases, with their true causes and effective treatments, than I had ever dreamed possible. A new layer on the "onion" of human pathology seemed to reveal itself, and I felt that I had been blessed to have it revealed to me. Certainly, there is always a greater comprehension to be had on any subject, but the results of toxin removal in improving otherwise totally unresponsive disease processes could not be ignored. It was just very difficult to believe that I was privileged enough to be given therapeutic insights largely unknown to most of my peers. My own professional strengths had always been in clinical medicine. Recognizing when sick people got better was well within my capabilities. Denying that such improvements were taking place was not a possibility. If a relentlessly progressive and incurable affliction was suddenly stabilizing and even improving, then I needed to know everything that could be known about why and how such a thing was happening. Where the pursuit of such information would lead was not a concern.

PART I

Metabolic Consequences of Dental Toxicity

1

Autoimmune Disease—An Overview

Autoimmune diseases can be quite varied in their clinical manifestations, but there is a definite family resemblance when you look at the causes and effects (or results) of the diseases. Examples of a few autoimmune disturbances are multiple sclerosis, Lou Gehrig's disease, systemic lupus erythematosus, and some forms of arthritis.

The common denominator among these diseases is that your immune system is somehow stimulated or provoked into attacking your own tissue. Normally, there are immune markers on your tissue that keep this from occurring. Your immune system can differentiate your tissue from foreign invaders, and there is no chance of "friendly fire" from within.

The white blood cells of your immune system are trained to operate a sophisticated surveillance program. Each day almost every cell in your body is "examined" by your immune system for cellular integrity. By this mechanism, dead and dying cells are eliminated, and new invaders are also discovered and eliminated. Almost all of your cells have a personal code marked on their external surfaces. These codes could be considered the license plates for your cells. When the plate is present, that cell is classified as a "self" cell. When this plate is altered or absent, however, the cell is identified as "nonself," and the immune system proceeds to remove it.

When this alteration of cellular surface occurs in a sick or dying cell, the immune systems performs a vital function in cleaning up the entire body and maintaining a healthy internal environment. However, in the case of autoimmune disease, the immune system is attacking cells that have been wrongly tagged. The immune system is still doing its job, although it has been deluded into attacking the wrong cells.

The heavy metals used in dentistry are some of the agents that cause cellular changes, which result in this chronic misidentification by the immune system. Mercury is especially effective in this task. On attaching to the cell membrane, enough physical change takes place that the cell is then recognized as "nonself," and the immune system proceeds with its cleanup function.

Mercury is so efficient in creating autoimmune responses that it is routinely used in university research animal studies involving autoimmune disease. Read the abstracts of scientific articles on autoimmune disease research, and you will often find mercuric chloride or a similar compound administered to the animals to generate the autoimmune response to be studied.

Where mercury attacks is somewhat dependent on a person's genetically "weak link." Autoimmune diseases are a result of a genetic predisposition plus an environmental exposure. If you have such a susceptibility and you are exposed to mercury from your fillings, you could well be a candidate for an autoimmune disease. For example, when mercury attacks the nervous system, there are a variety of problems that can result, ranging from minor tremors and numbness of body parts to epilepsy, multiple sclerosis, or other pronounced neurological diseases.

When mercury combines with hormones, inefficient or misdirected performance will often result. Hashimoto's thyroiditis is one good example of a hormonal derangement commonly attributed to an "unknown" autoimmune etiology. Low body temperature is one simple example of thyroid interference by mercury, and such a problem can lessen within days of proper amalgam removal and replacement with compatible materials. Diabetes or mild elevations of blood sugar can result from an autoimmune process initiated by mercury's attack on the pancreas.

Lupus is an especially good autoimmune disease for demonstrating the effect of amalgam on disease activity. Lupus will typically be monitored by a host of tests, most prominently the antinuclear antibody (ANA) test. Tests for this antibody give an indication of the ongoing level of autoimmune activity and disease severity. We have consistently seen statistically significant drops in the titers, or amounts of antibody, in patients undergoing dental revision with amalgam removal.

Even though many of these autoimmune conditions can be improved or even rarely reversed by removal of the offending fillings, a much better approach would be to avoid the dental toxicity and lessen the chance of contracting the diseases in the first place. Remember that you are in control, but only when you are completely informed.

References for this Chapter

Dixon, Robert L., ed. 1985. *Immunology and Immunopharmacology*. Target Organ Toxicology Series. New York: Raven Press.

Hood, L. E., I. L. Weissman, W. B. Wood, J. H. Wilson. 1984. *Immunology*. 2d Ed. Redwood City, Calif.: Benjamin/Cummings Pub.

2

Birth Defects

The Greatest Joy—Jeopardized

"So you're going to have a baby. What do you want, a boy or a girl?"

"A healthy baby more than anything else."

This should be a fairy tale from here on, but it can be a nightmare. A preventable nightmare, fortunately—for the informed.

The uninformed, on the other hand, can create birth defects in their own children in a completely inadvertent fashion. With total unawareness and complete permission, they can walk into a dental office, have their teeth filled, and walk away with a mouth perfectly designed to slowly release potent toxins into their bodies and across their placental barriers.

Official Warning

California, in a brave step forward, is the first state to admit that it knows one of the causes of birth defects. What is more significant, California is willing to take the position of informing potential parents of the presence of this defect-causing toxin. This toxin is mercury.

Only a few years ago science stated that there were only two causes of birth defects: exposures to X-rays, and exposures to mercury. Now there are many new chemicals that can produce birth defects, but the old causes remain. However, X-ray machines are easy to spot, but we probably won't spot the mercury vapor insidiously and incessantly emanating from our amalgam fillings.

For this reason, resisting 160 years of conventional dentistry, some brave people in California were willing to help the world identify the major source of mercury contamination in humans—the mercury amalgam filling. According to California's Proposition 65, passed almost a decade ago, anyone who exposes someone else to a material that can cause cancer, birth defects, or reproductive harm must inform the person to be exposed prior to the exposure. The exposure itself is not banned. However, the ability to secretly expose is banned. The catch phrase is "disclosure before exposure." As a result of this desire on the part of the state to protect the people of California, every dentist in California now has to display the following sign:

WARNING

This office uses amalgam filling materials which contain and expose you to a chemical known to the State of California to cause birth defects and other reproductive harm. Please consult your dentist for more information.

As straightforward as this warning is, the dental board in California nevertheless threatens dentists with loss of their licenses if they say anything derogatory about mercury amalgam fillings in advising and counseling their patients. This threat to licensure is very real, as several outspoken dentists have lost their licenses in the past few years. As a further threat to the nonconforming dentist, the Division of Legal Affairs of the American Dental Association (ADA) inflicts further constraints. A dentist cannot mention that mercury is the most poisonous natural element on the planet (an unchallenged scientific statement) and then suggest the removal of any amalgam fillings. Specifically, the dentist cannot remove mercury fillings "for the alleged purpose of removing toxic substances from the body, when such treatment is performed solely at the recommendation or suggestion of the dentist." Such a suggestion is further deemed "improper and unethical." If found guilty of being conscientious and giving honest counsel to the patient about the known dangers of mercury, the dentist faces unending harassment and legal challenges in the continuing practice of dentistry, potentially resulting in the loss of his or her dental license. The dentist is forced to be an unwilling and silent co-conspirator in the poisoning of his or her patients.

In Colorado, Administrative Law Judge Nancy Connick even went so far as to write in one of her rulings that Colorado *patients* who are aware of the toxicity of mercury and request its removal are also liable for fine and imprisonment. Although this is not Colorado law, this enormous attempt to overreach by a prominent member of the judiciary system should scare the daylights out of anyone who thinks there exists an unchallenged right to protect self and family.

Firsthand Experience

Witnessing the cause of a birth defect by mercury is not very pleasant, but it is enlightening. A good example of this follows.

One day two separate containers in a chemistry laboratory fell and broke within minutes of each other. Mercury was running all over the place. The clean-up crew had to be summoned. The next day I was called.

"Huggins?"

"Yeah, this is Huggins."

"Could you look into something for me—as a favor? We got a mercury problem."

"Sure. What's the story?"

After going on for a while, he finally ended up: "and today we have two students staying home because of strange illnesses."

"Got any blood results?"

"White cell count of 16,000 with over two-thirds of the PMNs severely multinucleated. Get your attention?"

"I'd say so."

After a couple of weeks things had calmed down a bit, and the students appeared to have normalized. Everything was forgotten. But another call came the week later.

"Hug?"

"You sound concerned. What's up?"

"She's pregnant."

"The, ah . . ."

"That's right, one of the students who got a little sick after the mercury spill."

"How far along?"

"Seven weeks at the time of the exposure. Didn't know she was pregnant back then. She'd miss a period sometimes for no good reason, so she had no reason to know."

"So we're in the first trimester."

"Yep. The whole brain development period."

That happened on day number two of a seminar that I was teaching to doctors and dentists on the topic of mercury toxicity. I had opened the session this way:

"Okay, ladies and gentlemen, let me share something with you that goes with the territory of working in the field of mercury toxicity. There was a mercury spill." Then I told the story. "Now, what would you do if you were the attending doctor? What would you do if you were the young lady who is pregnant? What would you say if you were her husband?"

"By God, if she was my daughter, she'd have an abortion," bellowed the gruff voice of a male dental school professor.

"'By God,'" echoed a female dental school professor. "Does that mean you're playing God? It sure sounds that way to me."

"Me, too," chimed in a dentist's wife. "Do you think you have a right to play God this time, too? We're not in class."

Good-hearted laughter then resounded from the several of us who knew the first professor and were very familiar with his teaching techniques.

"Now wait a minute," said a dentist's wife who had not yet uttered a word during the seminar. "Our son and his wife had a child with birth defects, and she left him after two years. Her folks won't foot any of the massive bills, and our son will probably spend the rest of his life working to pay those bills, along with the new ones accumulating every week. He will probably never have a life of his own. Neither will his daughter. She isn't aware of much of anything. Try living that kind of life for a year or two before you make a judgment."

"This is not a judgment; it's about what is right," added a physician. "Yes, I am Catholic, but that doesn't have anything to do with it. Regardless of religion, any child has a right to try for life and live it, win or lose."

"I've treated many of these kids in the school," the gruff dental professor again spoke, and everyone let him have the floor. "Med school sends them over. Cleft lip, cleft palate, some cleft chest and heart—those generally don't make it. And I can tell you it ain't no fun for anyone. And mercury can cause any of them defects. I got three kids—all boys. They're teenagers now. I gotta tell you, they're all normal brats, and even being healthy they were tough enough to raise. I love 'em, and I guarantee you I wouldn't wish birth defects on my worst enemy. And I got some."

Is there a compromise here? Hardly. But what about the pregnant college student who was exposed early in her pregnancy to spilled mercury in the laboratory? What was her opinion about all of this? Not surprisingly, the young lady elected to keep the pregnancy. She delivered a beautiful eight-pound baby girl, pronounced by the delivering physician as being perfectly healthy after the first examination.

Three minutes later, the baby had her first seizure.

Can mercury-caused birth defects be prevented? In some cases, yes. But, to prevent them, you have to know something about how they originate. In researching an earlier book, *Why Raise Ugly Kids,* I first learned some unsettling truths about birth defects and their causes. Sources of mercury exposure, the effects of such exposure on parental fertility, the biological action of mercury, the defense (if any) provided by the placental barrier against invading mercury, and the consequences of mercury's interference in normal development all needed to be considered together. The picture was as fascinating as it was disturbing.

Dental Sources of Mercury

According to Lars Frieberg, M.D., Ph.D., former head of toxicology of the World Health Organization, silver mercury amalgam fillings are the largest single source of mercury exposure in the worldwide population. Called "silver fillings" due to their initial shiny appearance, amalgam is made from powders of copper, tin, silver, and zinc mixed with approximately 50% liquid elemental mercury.

The chemistry of the setting of silver mercury amalgam after it is placed in the mouth is complex, incompletely understood, and people are told by the dental association that a stable compound has been formed as a result of the setting process. The ADA even reports that mercury is "tightly bound" within the compound.

I asked toxicologist Joe Levisky what the best way to analyze the amount of mercury in a filling might be, and he replied, "Weigh the filling, heat it, and weigh it again. The difference is the amount of mercury. This is probably the simplest and most accurate method." If simply heating amalgam causes it to release all of its mercury, it really isn't tightly bound.

Although electron microscopes have been used to demonstrate tiny droplets of mercury on the surface of amalgams, it doesn't take really high magnification to demonstrate the release of mercury. This ease of release makes us question the dental community's comments about mercury being "rendered harmless" and "inert" while in the mouth, even though dentistry does not argue that mercury is hazardous waste if it is removed from the mouth.

After implantation in your teeth, and for an indefinite period of time, silver mercury fillings outgas readily detectable amounts of mercury vapor. This is in the range of 1 to 50 micrograms of mercury per cubic meter of air. Even one microgram of mercury is adequate to destroy any type of cell in the body, especially nerve tissue. Two generally accepted facts about mercury and amalgam are that mercury escapes at a rate of one microgram per surface of filling per day, and that mercury will accumulate in tissues from low-dose chronic exposure. Most amalgams have multiple surfaces as defined here, so a mouthful of amalgam fillings can result in a substantial amount of mercury vapor.

You may think that a chronic accumulation of even this low a dosage of something as toxic as mercury is bad enough, but this refers only to a mouth at rest. How much of the time is a mouth at rest? After only ten minutes of gum chewing, Dr. Carl Svare of the Ohio State School of Dentistry measured an average increase in mercury release of 15.6 times more than during the resting state in test subjects. That converts to a 1,560% increase in mercury release. Chewing your food well is a vital element in achieving good health, but the benefit of thorough chewing is less clear-cut when your mouth is full of amalgam.

Brune examined the new state-of-the-art amalgams called "high-copper" amalgams. He found that the newer fillings (post-1976) emit up to 50 times more mercury than the earlier, conventional amalgam fillings. That means that every new high-copper amalgam filling placed today can have the effective toxic equivalent of placing fifty of the older amalgam fillings.

If other fillings are in the mouth, such as gold crowns, nickel crowns, and removable bridges or braces, the mercury emission further increases from the amalgam. This is due to the electrical current generated by the presence of dissimilar metals being present in an electrolyte such as saliva.

The chemical nature of foods can also affect the rate of release of mercury from amalgam. Of course, the very act of chewing the food will have its own accelerating effect on mercury release, but the effect will be even further pronounced if the food is chemically active. Vinegar-and-oil dressing for your salad might be fine for the digestion, but the acidic nature of the vinegar will also promote mercury release from fillings. Many other foods can possess varying degrees of acidic properties.

Heat will also reliably increase the rate of escape of mercury vapor from amalgam fillings. One time when we had the mercury vapor detector handy and an ABC-TV camera was rolling, we gave a volunteer two ounces of hot water to drink. The volunteer downed the water in one gulp, rather than prolonging the exposure through slow sipping. Nevertheless, the vapor detector above his amalgams moved from 3 micrograms to over 500 micrograms by ten seconds after the hot drink was swallowed.

What should be most apparent from these examples is that silver mercury fillings are not very stable. These fillings emit mercury vapor in their resting state, and their emission rate accelerates dramatically after minimal mechanical, chemical, and temperature stimulations. Combined with the massive outgassing characteristics of the high-copper amalgam, the daily mercury exposure from any number of amalgams cannot be dismissed as minimal.

Mercury's Effects on Fertility

Who is responsible for fertilization? Both parents, of course. And who is responsible for birth defects? Again, both parents. Reproductive harm reflects damage to the reproductive system in either males or females.

Many women cannot even reach the first step of conception. This could actually be considered a form of a birth defect in itself, but it is better known as "reproductive failure." Both ovaries and testes have been found to be sites of mercury accumulation. When the human egg is exposed to mercury, it sometimes loses its ability to become implanted in the wall of the uterus, even if the fertilization process was successful.

Mercury can also directly interfere with the male's ability to manufacture sperm. Low sperm counts can be attributed to mercury toxicity in some patients. In addition, mercury can directly inhibit the cellular ability to reproduce the genetic code called DNA in the sperm itself. Here the resulting birth defect can occur at the "half-cell" level, prior even to fertilization. This would be an example of a strictly male contribution to defective development after fertilization.

Certain enzymes are necessary for proper sperm development. Not surprising, mercury can slow down the reactions of these enzymes to the point that they cannot provide the DNA interconnections at the speed necessary to complete the proper formation of healthy sperm.

Apparently, then, a birth defect can originate from the contribution of either the male or the female partner. The female tends to typically assume the burden of an undesirable outcome, since the developing fetus spends 100% of its time in the female environment, and any toxic influences from the female will have direct effects on fetal development. However, multiple mechanisms of preconception exposure to mercury and other toxicity can implicate either parent in defective fetal development.

Chromosome Damage from Mercury

Birth defects are frequently the result of interference with the duplication of our genetic template. We have a code that is copied enough to create the thirty or so trillion cells that make up an adult human body. Within our genetic code, called DNA, there are 23 pairs of chromosomes, giving a total of 46. We obtain one set of 23 from each parent.

Mercury has been found to produce "aberrant chromosome numbers." This means that, instead of 46 chromosomes, a child with a birth defect might have 45 or 47 chromosomes. Examples of such aberrancy are seen in Down's syndrome and Klinefelter's syndrome. A larger deviation than one chromosome from the 46 total will often result in death of the fetus, followed by resorption or spontaneous abortion. Mercury at as low a dosage as one tenth of a part per million can produce breaks in chromosomes. If this break occurs in an early-enough stage of organ development, focusing on a critical area like the heart or brain, a spontaneous abortion will often terminate this pregnancy as well.

Researcher Verschaeve found that there was a significant correlation between the amount of mercury in the blood and the number of chromosomal aberrations. Other papers have shown that the amount of mercury in the blood is directly related to the number of mercury fillings in that person. Mercury is also found to accumulate in the fetus at substantially higher levels, up to thirty times more, than it does in its mother.

After fertilization, the one fertilized cell must duplicate itself many billions of times, a process called mitosis. This process involves the progressive division of a cell, with a doubling in number every time the division takes place. As cell division continues, and specific enzymes exert their influence, cellular "split-offs" occur, with resultant cellular specializations. These specializations manifest as heart, liver, kidney, muscle, bone, and other tissues. If any mercury atoms are present at any one of these initial cell division points, an alteration of the final tissue pattern or formation can occur. Further, if this mercury-altered cell manages to survive, a "mutant" cell will have been formed. And if the ability to adequately duplicate itself has not been affected as well, such a cell can directly contribute to a defective tissue or organ. Many times this alteration is not noticed at birth, but, when present, it can be passed on to succeeding generations as a genetic "family trait." Such a trait cannot be stopped as long as the new adults continue to have their own families.

So chromosomes can be visualized as the instructors of our genetic templates, directing the formation of a new human being. Therefore, any interference in chromosome design can be anticipated to alter the final product. Mercury can provide this interference, which can result in birth defects.

The Placental Barrier

The concept of a placental barrier doesn't really apply when measuring the toxicity of mercury. In fact, mercury, in any of its chemical forms, can cross any barrier or cell membrane in the body. The placenta can afford a measure of protection to the fetus when acutely exposed to inorganic mercury, but this protection will only last from a few minutes to no more than an hour. Methylmercury, especially from fish and other seafood, passes through the barrier the fastest. Unfortunately, this form of mercury probably does the most damage—especially to the developing brain and nervous system. Only recently have public health authorities begun to address this problem, actually advising the minimization of fish consumption from specified U.S. waters by pregnant women.

Karp and Gale found that mercury alters the activities of five different human enzymes that control activities in the placenta. One of these, cytochrome C oxidase, is of great significance, for it is active in the production of ATP, the primary energy source for all biological activity in our cells. The alteration of these placental enzymes was found to result in fetal kidney damage, mental retardation, defects in the fetal chest wall, cleft palate, and abnormal heart alterations.

One thing is for sure: The term "barrier" does not apply to mercury.

Consequences of Fetal Exposure to Mercury

Kuntz found that the amount of mercury in the blood of the mother correlated with the number of amalgam fillings in her mouth. Also, some fetal tissues (such as the red blood cells) will reliably concentrate mercury in higher levels than the mothers' tissues. Kuntz further reported that stillborn infants had higher levels of mercury than live children, and those levels were higher than their mothers'. Within this range of seemingly unaffected live births and stillborn births will be found the mercury-exposed babies with birth defects. Let's look at the specifics of some of these mercury-induced birth defects.

In studying the results of mercury exposure in the brain, Choi found that mercury had a more selective than general effect. He found that mercury exposure in the brain produced new pathways of development. Instead of nerves growing from the brain to the places genetically pre-determined to create a hookup, the presence of mercury would create a "deranged alignment of neurons." This happened in both the cerebrum and cerebellum portions of the brain. The cerebrum is the so-called intellectual portion of the brain that processes memory and thought. The cerebellum is that part of the brain that coordinates rapid muscle activities, although it does have to interact with the cerebrum to produce coordinated muscle activity. Thus, these segments of the brain are not totally autonomous.

Choi examined the cerebral cortex, which is the "central clearinghouse" for directing messages. The cerebrum is essential for correcting errant messages on the spot. For example, if you were riding a bicycle in a circle, there would have to be compensating shifts in weight and steering on a continual basis. Similarly, playing a piano, typing, or playing tennis would require this same type of constant redirection of impulses. This corresponds well with my observation when examining the mouths of Olympic hopefuls at the Olympic Center here in Colorado Springs. Some had one or two amalgams. A rare athlete had more than two. Most had none.

Another researcher, Khera, noted that in animals where most of the litter died due to mercury exposure, those that did survive had a reduced number of neurons. These were the nerve cells in the cerebellum, the coordination center. If the hookups are altered and the number of neurons is reduced, it is easy to see why coordination is difficult in many children with birth defects. Excessive blockage of neural impulses can result in paralysis, but most often a substantial blockage of these impulses will result in spastic action of the affected muscles.

My own observation has been that visual alterations are probably the most common alteration of early mercury exposure. Astigmatism can result from a relatively minor mercury exposure. Mercury can readily be seen as black areas in the retina, thought by many to be a normal variant resulting from a stretching of the retina that reveals the underlying epithelium. This is often concentrated around the optic disc as a crescent-shaped black or darkened area. These areas have been noted to lighten, coincident with the improvement of vision, after the removal of amalgam.

In animal studies, the fetal retina demonstrated damage after the mother's single mercury exposure. Further, the damage was not apparent at birth. It was not until adulthood that the impaired process of visual stimulation was noted. Specifically, exposures to mercury immediately before or after birth can produce a loss of neurons in *all* areas of the visual cortex. This cortex is the area that is critical for our primary vision. Although many other areas of the brain are involved in mercury toxicity, none is as consistently damaged as those areas involving sight.

Some birth defects, like conjoined Siamese twins, are easy to identify. Now researchers are finding defects that were actually present at birth, but not identified until much later in life. Chang mentions that minute amounts of mercury, incapable of producing a grossly apparent birth defect, can create "cellular dysfunction," going undetected for decades until another stress compromises an organ function. A disease of "unknown origin" can then become manifest.

One reason for this delayed action is that the developing brain has many compensatory mechanisms that allow it to handle normal activities for even ten or more years and escape detection at birth. In some cases the abnormal responses may be identified earlier when a certain predictable milestone in normal development is delayed in onset. Such milestones include the timing and taking of the first step or the first word, the use of the potty, or the cutting of the first tooth. Delays in these developments have been noted in children of mercury-exposed mothers. Typically, the mothers of these children had no observable symptoms of toxicity whatsoever.

The challenges that finally produce symptoms later in life can assume many forms. Ingesting lead or mercury from paint on the wall, living near a toxic waste dump, or having orthodontic braces and high-copper amalgams can all tip the scales in favor of overt clinical toxicity. The brain finally fails in its ability to further accommodate to and compensate for the additional stresses and insults. This has led many researchers to identify many behavioral abnormalities as birth defects.

Behavioral abnormalities can become manifest well before congenital brain malformations are produced by mercury. Marlowe added a level of complexity to this observation by noting the combined effects of multiple metal exposures. In dentistry, amalgam fillings contain five toxic metals: copper, tin, silver, zinc, and mercury. (Certain organic compounds derived from some of these elements can be beneficial and nutritive, and they should not be confused with these inorganic toxic compounds.) Teeth braces typically contain nickel, chromium, and cobalt. Marlowe used a scale called the WPBIC to measure such behaviors or traits as acting-out, withdrawal, distractibility, disturbance in peer relations, and immaturity. He concluded that exposure to multiple metals was not merely additive in the cumulative toxicity. Rather, he found that the presence of multiple toxic metals caused substantial mutual magnification of the others' toxic effects.

In our research using planaria (a small aquatic creature that is relatively sensitive to toxins—the "canary in the mine" of the water kingdom) and human white blood cells, we examined this toxin magnification phenomenon. A small concentration of mercury added to either white blood cells (lymphocytes) or planaria would kill a certain percentage of them. The same was true of copper. But add the two toxins together and the result was magnified. The total kill substantially exceeded the numbers seen with the toxins individually administered then added together. (See Figure 1 on the following page.)

Another animal researcher, D. C. Rice, studied the impact of mercury exposure before and shortly after birth. He observed the development of pronounced behavioral changes as the animals grew. He suggested a practical approach to assessing mercury toxicity on animal or human development. His proposal was that behavioral alterations might be a better indicator of mercury toxicity than any clinical evidence of gross birth defects and organ pathology, a true "functionalistic" approach.

Although mercury has many well-established toxic effects early in pregnancy, its toxicity is not limited to this period. Rice found that cerebral palsy from mercury exposure occurs only when that exposure is during the last three months of pregnancy. Choi also studied cerebral palsy. He stated that miniscule doses of mercury that produced no signs or symptoms within the initial months of exposure could nevertheless result in the development of cerebral palsy and progressive mental retardation years later. His findings indicated that the nervous system seemed to be increasingly susceptible to abnormal development as the child approached the early teen years.

Rice also associated "developmental retardation" with exposure to infinitesimal amounts of mercury.

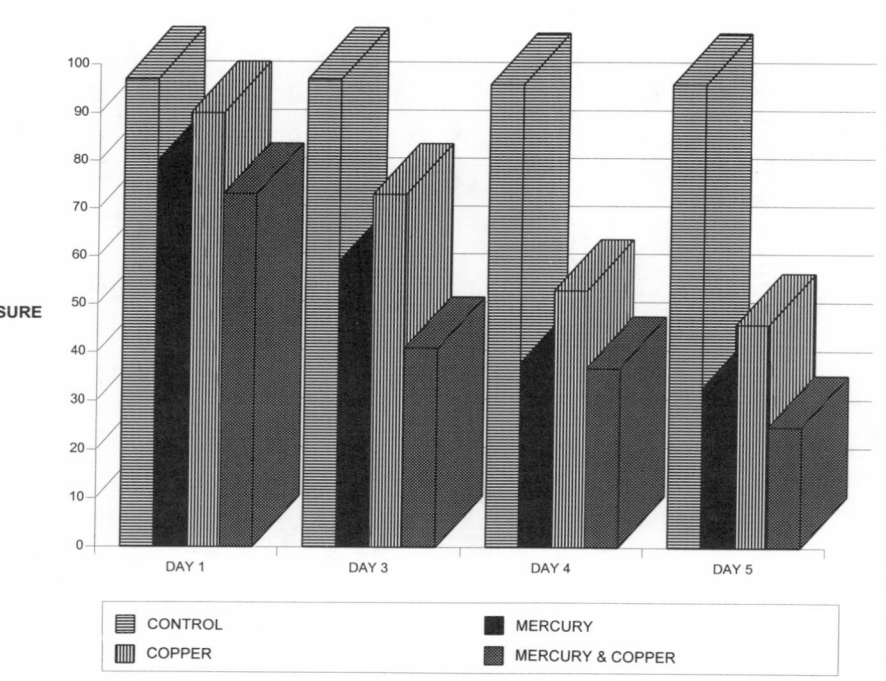

FIGURE 1: LYMPHOCYTE VIABILITY WHEN EXPOSED TO MERCURY & COPPER

% LIVE
AFTER EXPOSURE

CONTROL   MERCURY
COPPER   MERCURY & COPPER

This syndrome refers to the exaggerated muscle-nerve interplay that results in twitching and difficulty in handling objects without dropping them. This is also called "Minimal Brain Damage Syndrome."

To Recap

In addressing the topic of birth defects relative to mercury exposure, one should first address the initial exposure to mercury. In the dental office, this can come from the mother having silver-mercury (amalgam) fillings placed before or during pregnancy. Current amalgam fillings are likely to be the high-copper variety, outgassing up to 50 times more mercury vapor than the earlier version. Add to this the need to chew and the inevitable encounters with hot and acidic foods, and the mercury exposure escalates.

From the fillings, the mercury released can go directly into the lungs, or eventually into the intestinal tract. From either place, the mercury can end up in the bloodstream, then anywhere else in the body. Blood-borne mercury can easily cross the placental barrier. If there is an encounter with the ovaries, testes, or the uterus along the way, mercury can prevent fertilization from ever occurring. If fertilization does occur, interference at the early stages of development can alter chromosome formation and cellular replication. This can lead to related mutations and birth defects. Later interference, when the developing fetus is growing in the uterus, can lead to cleft palate, cleft lip, and myriad other developmental anomalies. Exposures during the later segments of development can lead to cerebral palsy, minimal brain dysfunction, and abnormal behavior patterns. If enough of these developmental interferences occur, the fetus can die. This results in a stillbirth, nature's way of eliminating many improper fetal developments before they proceed any further.

If a baby with a minimal exposure to mercury is born without obvious birth defects, what may you expect as time goes on? If mercury exposure is high enough to elicit a negative response, and the timing coincides with a major developmental event, there will be notable consequences. There may be a delay in the appearance of the typical "milestone" events such as the first step or the first word. Visual impairments, although initiated at this time, may not be noted until later, but muscular coordination may be notable. Microscopically, there can be a reduction in neuron count. Autopsy studies also point up deranged alignment of the neurons that did develop. In short, your child is retarded to some degree.

To Prevent

Not too many years ago, a pregnant female had to concern herself only with avoiding X-rays and mercury. Today the list of what should be avoided is nearly endless. Prescription drugs, over-the-counter drugs, illicit drugs, alcohol, and cigarettes carry warnings advising against their use or consumption during pregnancy. What is glaringly absent in such warnings is any concern for the male preparing to make his contribution to the upcoming pregnancy. For the good of the future infant, both prospective parents must be protected. While the following is expressed from the standpoint of mercury toxicity, other toxic exposures would follow the same rationale.

Dr. Louis Chang of the University of Arkansas asserts that, before pregnancy, both parents are comparably sensitive to mercury. However, after fertilization occurs, the mother becomes twice as sensitive as before, and the new fetus becomes four times more sensitive to mercury exposure than its mother. This makes the fetus eight times more sensitive than its father. This means that only one-eighth as much exposure to mercury by the fetus will damage it as much as a full dose to the father. Along with this, one must also consider that the fetal red blood cells will contain generally about 30% more mercury than the mother, even though the same blood supply is shared.

Planning for a baby is an important part of many cultures. Planning here refers to far more than the typical American preparation of buying a crib and stockpiling disposable diapers. Weston Price, D.D.S., in his well-researched book, *Nutrition and Physical Degeneration,* described what a "primitive" African colony would routinely do when a couple decided to wed. After informing the tribal counsel of their intentions, the couple was pronounced engaged, and the preparations for a healthy pregnancy were initiated. Remember that there was no effective birth control, and pregnancy was anticipated to occur soon after the marriage. Further, the entire tribe had strong interests in maintaining its overall strength through health, which ultimately affected the survival of the tribe as well. Both prospective parents were put on special diets to allow them to attain optimal health before conception could ever take place. These foods were supplied for a full six months before the marriage. By comparison to today's standards for optimal health, even being concerned about what a future parent ate a full six months before anticipated pregnancy sets a goal and a concern not even contemplated by modern medicine. Further, the diet chosen was rich in the nutrients known today to be necessary in the prevention of many birth defects. Primitive can be a very relative term.

In our clinic, "pre-preparation" was sometimes undertaken. When young couples want to do everything possible to ensure a healthy pregnancy, the use of blood testing can greatly facilitate the choice of the best foods. Certain food choices will nearly always be good for most people, but an improvement in certain blood chemistries is a reliable guide in ensuring the best choices have been made. Such chemistries can be used to determine the amount of carbohydrate, protein, and fat required to make up that individual's optimal diet.

If one lived in a toxin-free environment, the nutrition from a properly digested diet would be unchallenged as the most important factor in reaching good health and in preparing for the development of a new life. However, today's prospective parents are missing the most important step in assuring the health of their future children if their dental toxicity remains unaddressed. Potential birth defect-producing toxins abound in most mouths today. Mercury, nickel, root canals, and cavitations are all highly toxic, and leaving them in place before a planned pregnancy is not a certain indicator of an unhealthy baby, but they represent substantial and unnecessary risk factors contributing to birth defects.

Certainly, alcohol, cigarettes, and drugs of all kinds should be severely limited if they cannot be eliminated completely. Sometimes a certain medication is vital to maintaining the mother's good health, and a balancing of the interests of maternal and fetal health must be reached. Rationalizing any smoking or drinking during pregnancy is much more difficult.

Birth control, the typical modern precursor to the decision to finally have child, can be its own significant toxin exposure. Contraceptive creams and gels will often contain mercury. Even lubricated condoms can contain mercury. The uses and applications of mercury commercially would certainly never lead you to suspect that it is the most toxic nonradioactive heavy metal on the planet. In spermicidal preparations, mercury is almost uniformly the agent added to ensure that the sperm die. If use of an agent is so commonly accepted for a given purpose, the package need not even list it as a component. Combine this dosing of mercury with the mucosal membrane environment of the vagina, and you have another highly effective delivery system of mercury into the body. Further, what if the spermicide is only effective in damaging the sperm, but not preventing fertilization? This can be yet another mechanism for increasing the chance of a birth defect.

Research all of your options thoroughly before choosing how you want to prevent pregnancy. Think twice before considering vasectomy, too. Many studies indicate an increased incidence of premature cardiac death in such individuals. If you can't get satisfactory answers from your doctor, check out MEDLINE® and the World Wide Web for yourself. There is no longer any excuse for not getting all perspectives on any subject before making critical decisions. And there is more than one doctor out there who can help you. Be a complete participant in determining what happens to you and your future child.

When you are already pregnant and discovering this information for the first time, your choices are different still. Amalgam removal will certainly produce an increased mercury exposure while the fillings are being cut out. Is that mercury exposure more toxic than the exposure continually vaporizing off of the fillings? The stage of the pregnancy, the number of fillings, the quality of nutrition, and the availability of such treatments as intravenous vitamin C are all important considerations in deciding on amalgam removal and dental revision. There is no simple answer here. As always, you need to be optimally informed before making any decision.

For a comparison, let's look at an extreme case. Leukemia, covered in detail in Chapter 5, appears to be an overresponse of a healthy immune system to mercury exposure. White blood cell counts can shift rapidly and dramatically when a mercury challenge is suddenly removed, as when amalgam fillings are removed. A typical white cell count would only be between five and ten thousand. In some cases of very high white cell counts, a drop of as much as 50,000 cells per cubic millimeter of blood can occur within twenty-four hours of amalgam removal. If even a greater threat of damage were presented by more mercury exposure, one would anticipate that the white blood cells would go up. Conversely, a drop in this count suggests that the overall internal exposure to mercury has been significantly reduced, and that much less danger is anticipated by the white cells. Based on these observations, then, one could conclude that the fetus would sustain less of a toxic attack if amalgams were removed than if they were left in place. As always, be informed, and make you own best decision.

In the balancing decision between leaving amalgams alone and removing them, one must consider looking at everything that is available for patient (and fetus) protection. Certainly, large amounts of mercury vapor will be released from the high-speed drill, which hits amalgam at speeds in excess of 100,000 revolutions per minute. But measures exist to help minimize the toxic exposure. A rubber dam, which is a thin sheet of rubber (about the thickness of a balloon), can somewhat isolate the teeth and fillings from the rest of the mouth. The dam exposes the teeth through tiny holes, greatly reducing the amount of swallowed amalgam particles and the amount of mercury vapor exposed to the absorptive mucous membranes under the tongue.

Heat is primarily what causes the vaporization of mercury in the drilling out of amalgam. During the basic cutting procedures, the dental assistant can squirt additional water on the dental burr-amalgam interface with a syringe. Although the drill has its own continuous spray of water during the drilling process, the syringe supplies the extra water needed for adequate cooling of the amalgam. This cooling is the important factor in minimizing the amount of mercury vapor release.

Mercury vapor exposure can be further minimized with negative ion generators or charcoal filters in the dental operatory. Both ambient mercury vapor and amalgam particulate matter circulating in the air can be extracted in this manner. For mercury already absorbed into the body, intravenous vitamin C can be invaluable in minimizing the acute toxic effect. Ideally, vitamin C should be infused before, during, and immediately after the amalgam extraction process. Heavy-metal chelators, such as DMPS and DMSA, are not advised during pregnancy. In fact, much of the time they should just be avoided. Possible reasons why are covered in detail in Chapter 15, on detoxification.

Unfortunately, you will be exposed to hundreds of sources of mercury. There is still not a "healthy" regard for the toxicity of mercury in our society today. The best you can do is to know where the largest and most consistent exposure will be. The "big two" are, and remain, dental amalgam in your mouth and eating seafood. But always look for the lesser, but easily avoidable, mercury exposures. Mercury and mercury-containing solutions continue to be used to sterilize different medicaments. Many eye drops and contact lens wetting solutions have used thimerosal, a mercury-containing solution, in the past. Over the past ten years, many such solutions have finally started using alternative sterilizing agents. Always look for "mer" somewhere in the names of the ingredients on the labels of different solutions. *Mer*curochrome, *mer*thiolate, and thi*mer*osal would typically be such names. Even immunization shots will often contain mercury-based preservatives. Any solution, injectable or otherwise, should be suspect.

Seafood, especially fish, deserves a separate mention here. Sad to say, fish contain large amounts of mercury. Even worse, the mercury is in the form of methylmercury, a form of mercury up to 100 times more toxic clinically than the inorganic mercury vapor coming off the amalgam filling. We have already seen that the vapor is quite toxic before any chemical modifications are made to it.

Biologically speaking, there is no "safe" level of mercury. Zero exposure would unquestionably be the best level. However, mercury is so widespread in our society today that zero exposure levels are not realistic and effectively unattainable. For that reason, the "safe" level of mercury exposure was politically set at 0.5 parts per million. Anything over that (especially in fish) is illegal to sell for human consumption. One point zero part per million (1.0 ppm) is considered the "action level" at which "something" must be done. Selling certain types of fish for human consumption in some countries has actually been banned, due to the high mercury levels, but this concept is very difficult for people of commerce and the seafood industry to accept. For that matter, such organizations as the American Heart Association are still actively promoting diets high in fish and seafood. If a group of board-certified cardiologists is telling you to eat seafood and fish often and deliberately, it's hard to imagine that the exact opposite dietary advice could be the best advice.

In one state, the fish in a reservoir were alleged to contain excess mercury. The State Department of Public Health proceeded to study the situation, determining that there was mercury in that reservoir's fish, but that "the level was no higher than the rest of the fish in the state." If such an official declaration is comforting to you, consider that the mercury level in question here, the one that was "no higher than the rest of the fish in the state," was 1.62 parts per million. Remember that a huge percent of the world's food supply would be excluded and deemed inedible if the toxicity of ingested dietary mercury were given proper credence. Since the overall supply of food in the world remains short without the exclusion of seafood, it will be unlikely that politically deemed safe levels of mercury will ever exclude most seafood. But remain aware that if you are trying to optimize your health and prepare for a healthy pregnancy, seafood is not the wonderful food it is purported to be.

But people do eat seafood all the time and don't get sick. In fact, many people get weekly exposures to methylmercury in fish and show no obvious detrimental effect. They may even appear to be in the peak of good health until they contract cancer at age sixty or have their first heart attack at age fifty. Note that when amalgams are removed in those people having their weekly fish, secondary immune reactions can develop with prompt and dramatic negative clinical reactions, usually in the form of pronounced gastrointestinal distress, whenever mercury is later reintroduced in as large a dose as is seen in most fish meals. However, these immunoprotective reactions tend not to develop unless at least several months of seafood abstinence follow the amalgam removal, giving the immune system adequate time to recover the ability to vigilantly guard against mercury reintroduction. If you remain continually exposed to mercury from fish or amalgam fillings, your immune system will never heal to the point of being protective in this fashion.

Remember that, even if you aren't sure that taking these suggested steps will benefit your health, there are few steps that can be considered too extreme to assure your new baby of having its best opportunity for a healthy and happy life.

References for this Chapter

Bengt, R. G., et al. 1990. Foetal and maternal distribution of inhaled mercury vapour in pregnant mice. *Pharmacology and Toxicology* 67: 222-226.

Brune, D., et al. 1983. Gastrointestinal and in vitro release of copper cadmium, indium, mercury and zinc from conventional and copper-rich amalgams. *Scandinavian Journal of Dental Research* 91:66-7.

Burbacher, T. M. 1990. Methylmercury effects on the social behavior of macaca fascicularis infants. *Neurotoxicology and Teratology* 12: 65-71.

Chang, L. W. 1979. Pathological effects of mercury poisoning. *Biogeochemistry of Mercury in the Environment*. ed. J. O. Nriagu. Chapter 20. New York: Elsevier North-Holland Biomedical Press.

Chang, L. W., P. R. Wade. 1980. Prenatal and neonatal toxicology and pathology of heavy metals. *Advances in Pharmacology and Chemotherapy* vol. 17. San Diego: Academic Press.

Choi, B. H. 1989. The effects of methylmercury on the developing brain. *Progress in Neurobiology* 32:447-470.

Clarkson, T. W., et al. 1985. Reproductive and developmental toxicity of metals. *Scandinavian Journal of Work, Environment and Health* 11:145-154.

Cordier, S., et al. 1991. Paternal exposure to mercury and spontaneous abortions. *British Journal of Industrial Medicine* 48:375-381.

Goncharuk, G. A. 1977. Problems relating to occupational hygiene in women in production of mercury. *Gigiena Truda i Professionalnye Zabolevania* 5:17-20.

Uninformed Consent

Grandjean, P., et al. May/June 1992. Impact of maternal seafood diet on fetal exposure to mercury selenium and lead. *Archives of Environmental Health* vol. 47, no. 3.

Karp, W., T. F. Gale, et al. 1985. The effect of mercuric acetate on selected enzymes of maternal and fetal hamsters at different gestational ages. *Environmental Research* 36:351-358.

Khera, K. S. 1973. Teratogenic effects of methylmercury in the cat: Note on the use of this species as a model for teratogenicity studies. *Teratology* 8: 293-304.

Kuntz, W. D., R. M. Pitkin, A. W. Bosstrom, M. S. Hughes. June 15, 1982. Maternal and cord blood background mercury levels: A longitudinal surveillance. *American Journal of Obstetrics & Gynecology* 143:440-443.

Lee I. P., R. L. Dixon. 1975. Effects of mercury on spermatogenesis studies by velocity sedimentation cell separation and serial mating. *Journal of Pharmacology and Experimental Therapeutics* vol. 194, no. 1.

March, D. O., T. W. Clarkson. October 1987. Fetal methylmercury poisoning, relationship between concentration in strands of maternal hair and child effects. *Archives of Neurology* vol. 44.

Marlowe, M. J., Jacobs, J. Moon, C. Errera. 1984. Main and interacting effects of metal pollutants in emotionally disturbed children. *Monograph in Behavioral Disorders* 7:67-79. ed. R. B. Rutherford. Reston, Va.: Council for Children with Behavior Disorders.

Miller, R. M. September 1967. Prenatal origins of mental retardation. *Journal of Pediatrics* 71, no.3:455-458.

Price, Weston A. 1977. *Nutrition & Physical Degeneration.* 9th ed. Price-Pottenger Nutrition Foundation.

Rice, D. C., S. G. Gilbert. 1990. Effects of developmental exposure to methylmercury on spatial and temporal visual function in monkeys. *Toxicology and Applied Pharmacology* 102:151-163.

Sikorski, R., et al. 1987. Women in dental surgeries: Reproductive hazards in occupational exposure to metallic mercury. *International Archives of Occupational and Environmental Health* 59:551-557.

Spyker, J. M. August 1972. Subtle consequences of methylmercury exposure: Behavioral deviations in offspring of treated mothers. *Science* 177:621-623.

Svare, C. W., et al. September 1981. The effect of dental amalgams on mercury levels in expired air. *Journal of Dental Research* 60(9): 1668-71.

Verschaeve, L., et al. 1976. Genetic damage induced by occupationally low mercury exposure. *Environmental Research* 12:306-316.

3

Chronic Fatigue

Normally Sick?

Chronic fatigue is so common in our society today that many patients consider fatigue to be to the "normal" baseline state of health. Anyone who has enough energy to do anything but collapse in bed after a hard day's work must be regarded as supernormal, blessed with an unusually strong vitality. Over 90% of the patients that we saw in the center stated that chronic fatigue was one of their major problems. From the physiological standpoint, the syndrome of chronic fatigue could well be largely due to the toxicity of one or more dental materials. This presumption starts with an analysis of what is required in the production and transport of energy in the body.

Food for Thought

Oxygen is the prime requirement for all energy transfer in the body. It uses the same transport pathways in everyone. The air that we all breathe has an oxygen content of around 20% if the air quality is good. Part of it is absorbed into the bloodstream. Specifically, the hemoglobin binds the oxygen and carries it to all parts of the body. The transport to the tissues of the body takes place in the arteries of the body, which progressively branch into smaller vessels until capillaries are reached. The smallest capillaries actually require the red blood cells to undergo slight bending and distortion for them to effectively "flow" through the vessel. Delivery of oxygen to the tissues takes place primarily at this capillary stage. The capillaries gradually increase in size on the return trip to the lungs via the venous system.

The actual amount of oxygen that is potentially available to the tissues can be estimated by measuring the amount of hemoglobin in the blood. Generally, males have slightly higher hemoglobin counts than females. The level for males is around 15 grams of hemoglobin per 100 milliliters of blood; for females the level is about 13.4 grams.

The levels of hemoglobin in chronic fatigue patients can run below normal. Readings below 12 grams would clearly indicate inadequate blood levels of hemoglobin. While a few chronic fatigue patients did have hemoglobin levels below 12 grams, most of our patients, including the females, had levels of 14.5 or more! Some of the most fatigued patients had levels of 16 to 18 grams of hemoglobin.

The next stage in the evaluation of chronic fatigue patients with high levels of hemoglobin was often referral to a psychiatrist. The thinking here is that stress or an inability to cope with life was accounting for the overwhelming fatigue. Doctors become very uncomfortable dealing with people who they cannot help.

Hemoglobin can be likened to taxicabs in New York City. There are always lots of them around, giving the appearance that adequate transportation is readily available.

However, when most of those cabs have passengers, transportation is not readily available, even though cabs seem to be everywhere.

Hemoglobin has passenger seats for oxygen that are called binding sites. Each binding site is capable of binding to one oxygen molecule and transporting it to tissues that are low in oxygen. Oxygen jumps off the passenger seat and leaps to help the deprived tissue with little effort. Should mercury come alone, unlike oxygen, it jumps into the passenger seat, buckles up, and plans to stay there until the red blood cell is recycled. When enough mercury combines with these passenger seats on the hemoglobin, the body experiences chronic fatigue due to lack of oxygen transport, and may create more red blood cells in compensation. The compensation action thickens the blood, so increased numbers is not a good answer. That's like putting more cars on the freeway so traffic will move faster.

Another test sheds light on the paradox of low energy with high hemoglobin. The *oxyhemoglobin* test reflects how many oxygen molecules are actually *bound* to the hemoglobin molecules. In *venous* blood one should normally find a 65% to 70% saturation of oxygen remaining after the appropriate amount of oxygen has been utilized in meeting the normal demands of daily life. However, in the chronic fatigue patients the venous oxyhemoglobin levels would typically run from 18% to 40% saturation. Did this mean that chronic fatigue patients were using even *more* oxygen than other people? Not really, even though that may appear to be a logical conclusion. We found that the oxygen was never there in adequate amounts in the first place.

Hemoglobin has four binding sites on which to carry oxygen. But, oxygen is not the only thing that can bind to these sites. Mercury has a very strong affinity for attaching to these sites as well. The major difference is that oxygen can attach to hemoglobin and later release easily, as it is picked up in the lungs and later deposited in needy tissues. Mercury sets up a much more permanent relationship with the hemoglobin binding sites. Once mercury is bound to the hemoglobin in a red blood cell, it will typically stay there for the entire lifetime of that red blood cell. This is approximately 120 days.

Since one molecule of hemoglobin has four oxygen binding sites, then one atom of mercury will drop the oxygen-carrying capacity of that hemoglobin molecule by 25% after binding. If two atoms of mercury should attach, that hemoglobin molecule will have a 50% reduction of its oxygen-carrying capacity. Do these observations help to explain chronic fatigue?

The body has many different ways in which it can compensate. When you first look at any clinical situation or set of laboratory tests, you must always consider that the patient may already be undergoing several "layers" of compensation. When the transport of oxygen to the tissues is compromised by interference from mercury, the body will attempt to compensate in some way. Since the body cannot block the daily mercury doses released from the mercury amalgams, it will typically just make more red blood cells to compensate for this daily contamination.

Remember, though, that all of the new hemoglobin will still have to confront both oxygen and mercury as potential binders. If the mercury challenge was very limited, this compensatory increase in hemoglobin might even prevent the clinical picture of fatigue from appearing. If the challenge from amalgam continues daily in a relentless fashion, the compensatory rise in hemoglobin will still be overwhelmed by mercury, and chronic fatigue can result.

So, when one has higher than normal level of hemoglobin, the first assumption most clinicians will make is that the delivery of oxygen to the tissues could not possibly be a problem. Such an individual is likely to be told that there is no reasonable physical basis for feeling fatigued. Thus the psychiatrist.

Coors Data

To test this concept, a study was conducted on patients who had *only* mercury amalgam as a dental material in their mouths. Individuals with root canals, crowns, and braces were excluded, since our prior observations have indicated there are many different sources of dental toxicity. In fact, the vast majority of patients who came to our center had multiple sources of dental toxicity. We had strong opinions about what mercury amalgam could do by itself to the body chemistries, but we were lacking the hard data of a controlled, prospective study.

The Adolph Coors Foundation elected to fund just such a study. The Coors Study, as yet unpublished, looked at blood tests on people with *only* amalgam in their mouths. Testing was done four separate times on each patient in this study. Testing was done both before and after amalgam removal. Then amalgam was reinserted, and testing was done before and after the second removal of amalgam.

Serum biocompatibility testing was performed on all patients to choose a final replacement composite material that had the lowest predictable immunoreactivity available, minimizing any further immune challenges to the patients. The information from this testing indicated that typically a drop in hemoglobin occurred after amalgam removal. Apparently when amalgam is removed, the body's ability to eliminate contaminated hemoglobin also improves very quickly. As a result, the body rids itself of mercury-contaminated red blood cells more rapidly than would naturally occur in awaiting the expiration of the anticipated 120-day lifespan of the red blood cells. (See Figure 2.) Of the twenty-seven people tested in the study, twenty-two demonstrated a drop in their hemoglobin levels. Further note that 100% of patients who presented with hemoglobin levels greater than 14.5 grams dropped after amalgam removal (nineteen of nineteen). At first glance, this looks like amalgam placement improves hemoglobin levels, and removal makes them worse. However, numbers alone can be misleading if function is not also considered.

Logically, one could predict that those people whose hemoglobin levels had dropped would feel more fatigued than prior to amalgam removal. Yet this was decidedly *not* the case. *Everyone* felt some improvement in energy, and some individuals even felt far more energy than they had felt in years. The data supplied by the oxyhemoglobin levels held the explanation.

Venous oxyhemoglobin levels measure the actual percentage of oxygen saturation in the venous blood. They had risen dramatically. Of the twenty-seven patients, twenty had *increased* their oxygen saturations. Eleven had increased more than 20% of their oxygen saturation, and six had increased more than 30%. Eight of these patients had more than *doubled* their oxyhemoglobin levels! The mystery of why people with high hemoglobin levels could complain about fatigue was answered. The answer was not "It's all in your head."

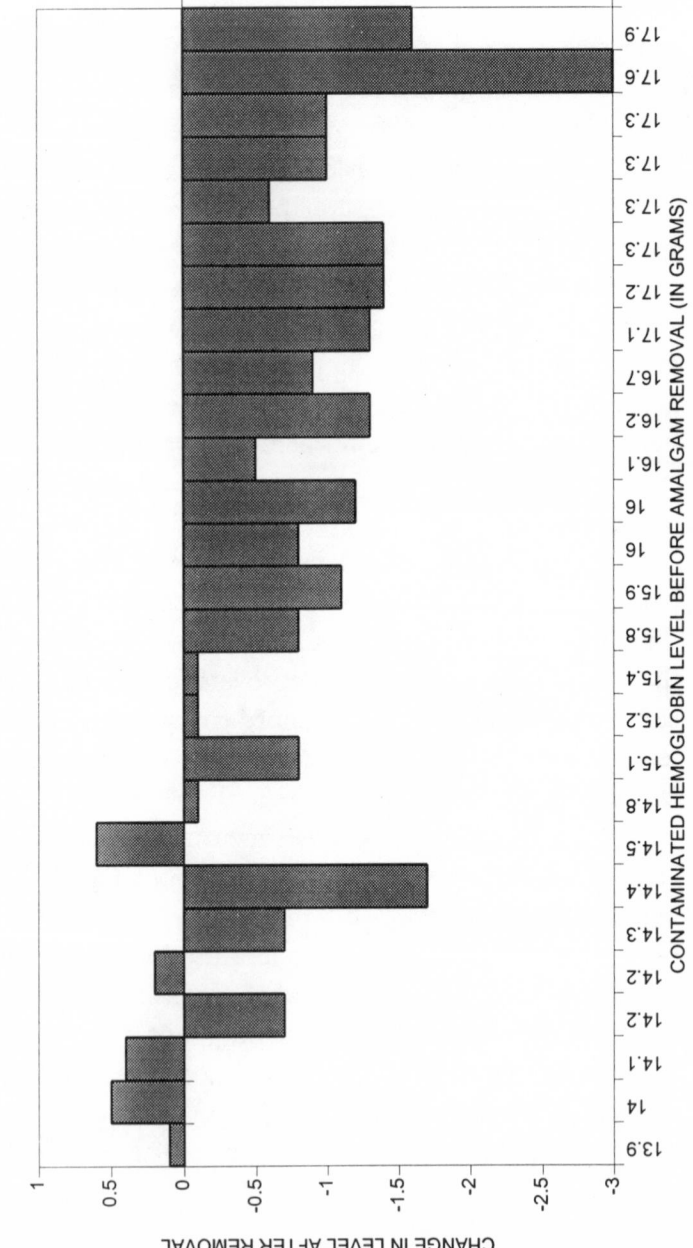

FIGURE 2: EFFECTS OF AMALGAM REMOVAL ON LEVELS OF CONTAMINATED HEMOGLOBIN

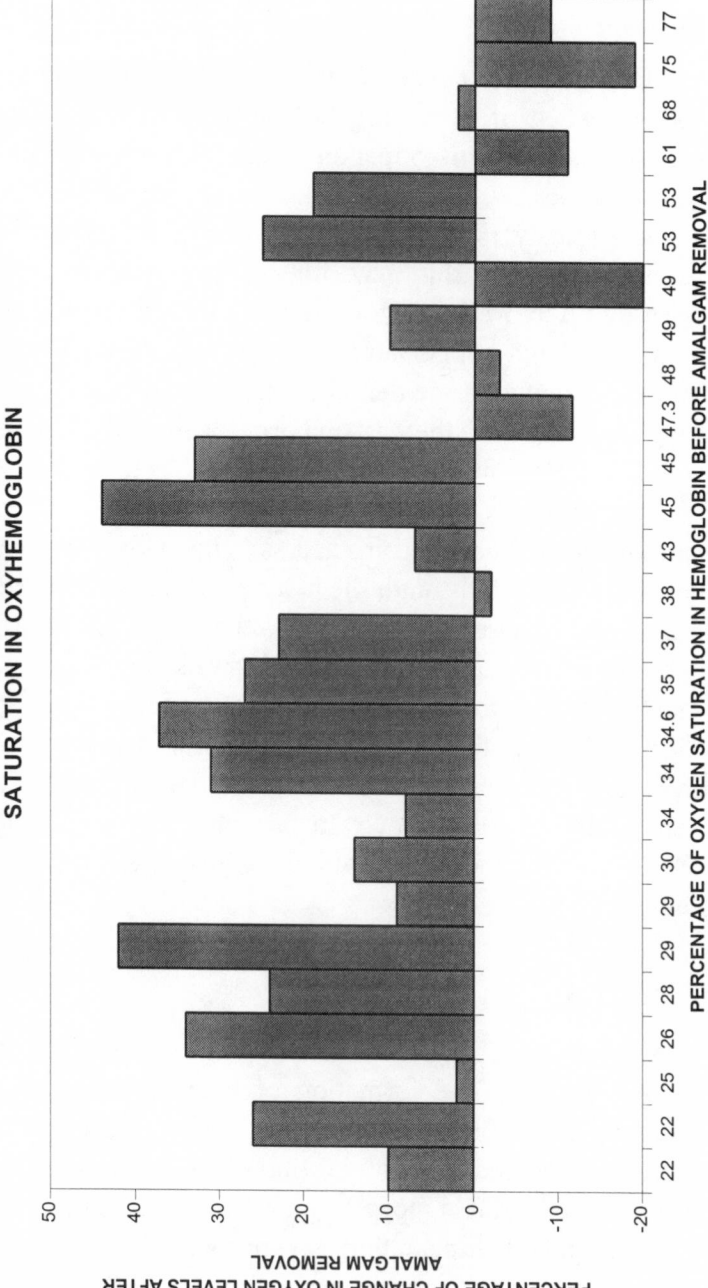

FIGURE 3: EFFECTS OF AMALGAM REMOVAL ON OXYGEN SATURATION IN OXYHEMOGLOBIN

Ready Mercury Sources

"Conventional" amalgam was routinely placed until the 1970s, when it was largely replaced by the new, state-of-the-art high-copper amalgam. This material substantially increased the percentage of copper in the new preparation over the old one. However, according to researcher Brune, this new 30% copper-mercury alloy released up to *50 times* more mercury than conventional amalgam. High-copper amalgam was well received and quickly accepted in the dental community. By the beginning of the 1990s, the vast majority of mercury fillings placed were of this high-copper variety.

Mercury vapor escaping from amalgam is the primary form in which mercury gains access to the body. Mercury vapor is absorbed through the mucous membranes of the mouth and by direct inhalation into the lungs. The stomach and intestinal tract also absorb swallowed forms of mercury freshly formed from the highly reactive vapor in the mouth. All of these *portals of entry* allow mercury relatively direct access to the bloodstream, where binding to hemoglobin can take place. In fact, the majority of the mercury in the blood is contained within the red blood cells.

Porphyrin

Mercury has another mechanism for producing chronic fatigue. The formation of hemoglobin can be impaired by the presence of mercury. When this effect is present, increased amounts of one of the basic building blocks of hemoglobin, porphyrin, will be seen in the urine.

A simplified explanation is appropriate here. The chemical complexities can get much more involved, but the purpose here is to transmit a usable, understandable concept. Porphyrin can be considered a layered molecule. The first layer consists of eight carboxyl groups. Enzymes cut off the carboxyl fragments to eventually leave a core molecule known as "heme." Heme has two energy functions. One involves its attachment to globin to form the familiar hemoglobin that transports oxygen. The other function involves heme undergoing a transformation down a chemical cascade of enzymes called the *cytochrome oxidase system*. During the course of this latter transformation, molecules of adenosine triphosphate (ATP) are formed. ATP is the primary cellular energy source in all functioning cells. Almost all the energy in our bodies is derived from these two energy sources. The transformation of porphyrin into heme or ATP is an integral part of the formation of energy in our bodies. Mercury appears to create an interference in porphyrin metabolism; the result is an identifiable increase in the urine of porphyrin breakdown products in lieu of energy forms.

On the graph addressing urinary porphyrins, note that there are columns marked with 8, 7, 6, 5, and 4. Three, two, and one do not exist for practical purposes. Four through eight are the porphyrins commonly detected in sophisticated testing. For orientation, look first at the graph of the person who never had amalgams or any other dental materials in his mouth. Only 12 micrograms are measured and all of this in the 4-carboxyl column. This indicates that some spillage of porphyrin can still be considered a part of normal metabolism. A "normal" value of up to 300 micrograms for total porphyrins has been suggested by the laboratory industry. This "normal" range, calculated on a population already implanted with mercury amalgam suggests that loss of porphyrins is acceptable. Again, the

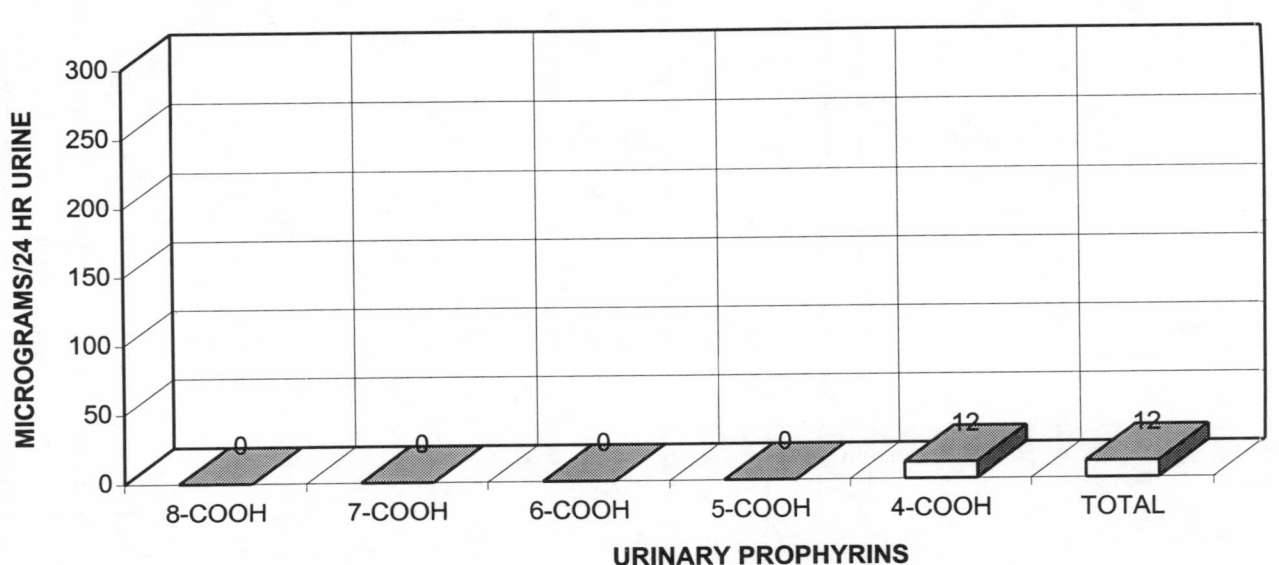

FIGURE 4: URINARY PORPHYRIN PROFILE ON A PATIENT WITH NO PREVIOUS DENTAL TREATMENT

Coors Study showed precisely what was influencing porphyrin excretion.

The following graph is from the Coors Study. Although all of the porphyrin measurements did not prove to be as dramatic as this one, this is nevertheless a good example of the effects of amalgam and its removal on urinary porphyrin excretion. Note the total level in segment one: 416 micrograms of total porphyrin were initially being excreted per twenty-four hours. After amalgam removal, the total excretion dropped to 35 micrograms. Reimplanting the amalgams increased the excretion to 149 micrograms. Final removal of the amalgams brought the level back down to 80 micrograms.

Note also that the reimplanted amalgams, to help preserve the teeth from unnecessary harm, were not nearly as large or with as much surface area as the initial amalgam fillings. Small fillings were reintroduced *into* the composite fillings that had been placed earlier and no drilling was done on the actual tooth structure.

In one multiple sclerosis patient, the total porphyrin excretion was 2100 micrograms. She had notable chronic fatigue symptoms. This is far above the accepted range of 300 micrograms. Also note that the toxic interferences affected *all* of the subclasses studied—4 through 8. This patient (not a Coors participant) also had crowns in addition to amalgams, so greater changes might be expected to occur upon the removal of this toxicity. Her levels of 4- and 5-carboxyl porphyrin dropped to zero, and the total porphyrin amount was only 200 micrograms after dental revision! A lot of metabolic energy was literally going down the toilet before this patient's mouth was properly restored.

When you remember the increase in oxyhemoglobin and the more efficient utilization of heme in the amalgam-free

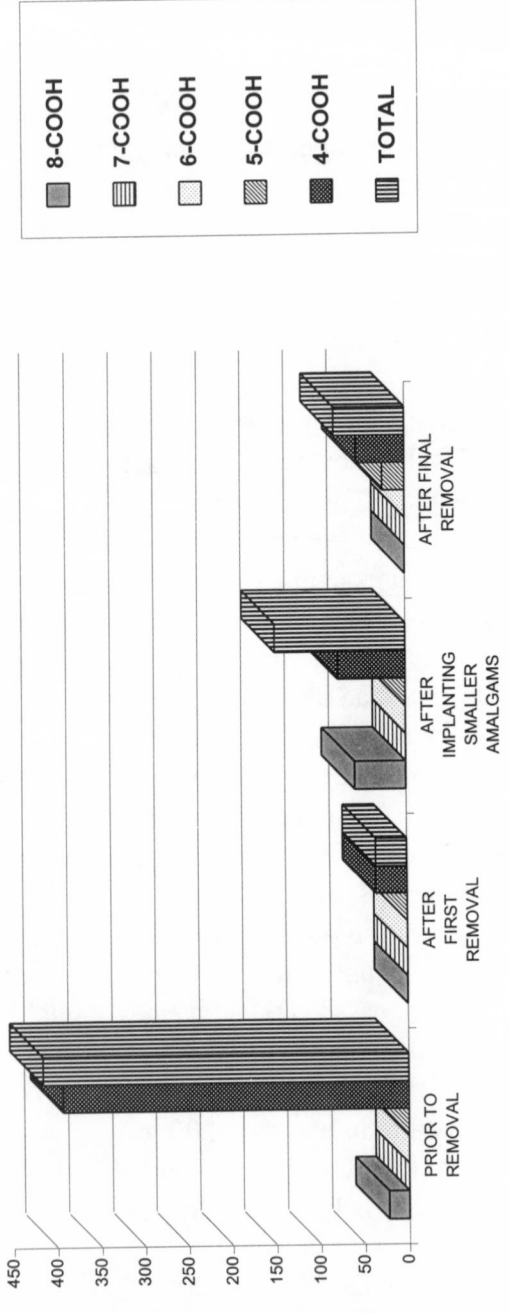

FIGURE 5: COORS STUDY ON RELATION OF PORPHYRIN LEVELS AND AMALGAM REMOVAL

FIGURE 6: PRE vs POST DENTAL URINARY PORPHYRINS
(MULTIPLE SCLEROSIS PATIENT WITH
AMALGAMS, CROWNS, AND CAVITATIONS)

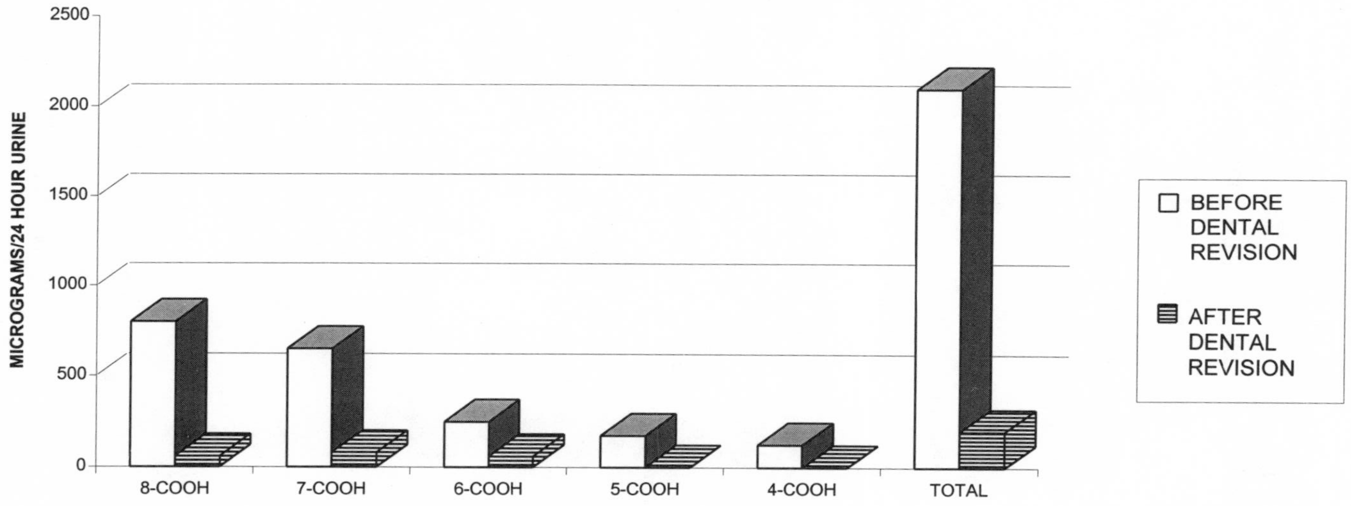

MICROGRAMS/24 HOUR URINE

2500 — 2000 — 1500 — 1000 — 500 — 0

8-COOH   7-COOH   6-COOH   5-COOH   4-COOH   TOTAL

□ BEFORE DENTAL REVISION

▤ AFTER DENTAL REVISION

patient, it becomes clear that mercury amalgam fillings, through more than one mechanism, may play a substantial role in the problem of chronic fatigue.

References for this Chapter

Beck, W. S., ed. 1985. *Hematology*. 4th ed. Cambridge, Mass.: The MIT Press.

Brune, D., et al. 1983. Gastrointestinal and in vitro release of copper cadmium, indium, mercury and zinc from conventional and copper-rich amalgams. *Scandinavian Journal of Dental Research* 91:66-71.

Coors Foundation, Adolph. Study of blood chemistry changes related to the presence and absence of amalgam (dental silver-mercury filling) in approximately 30 patients. Denver (unpublished data).

Woods, J. S., et al. 1991. Urinary porphyrin profiles as biomarkers of trace metal exposure and toxicity: Studies on urinary porphyrin excretion patterns in rats during prolonged exposure to methyl mercury. *Toxicology and Applied Pharmacology* 110:464-476.

4

Indigestion

Indigestion is a generic term that can refer to upset stomach, acid indigestion, food poisoning, diarrhea, or constipation. Indigestion primarily refers to poor food processing by the body. Let's look at the areas of indigestion observed over the past twenty-five years that appear dentally related.

Adults harbor several hundred species of so-called "friendly" bacteria in their stomachs and intestinal tracts that help digest carbohydrate, protein, and fat. Where did these friendlies come from?

When a child is born, its gastrointestinal tract is free from bacteria. As the child nurses, sucks its thumb, or otherwise experiences contact between its mouth and immediate environment, a common bacteria (Aerobacter) in the air mixes with the saliva and is swallowed. Strangely enough, on day four after birth, Aerobacter disappears and is instantly replaced with another bacteria. A few days later, other bacteria appear.

Where do all of these bacteria come from? Through a process called pleomorphism, many bacteria alter themselves in response to their immediate environment and become different bacteria. This is why the intestinal tract has so many different bacteria living within it. Differences occur in size, shape, and body functions. These changes in body function lead to differences in their personal biological wastes—and that is where some of our problems arise.

The metamorphosis of a butterfly is strongly analogous to the pleomorphism of these microscopic life forms. It starts out as a worm. The worm makes a cocoon and the worm later emerges as a butterfly. Quite a pleomorphic change in body form—from a lowly worm to a flying piece of art.

In the case of bacteria, as the stomach environment changes with the addition of new and different foods, some bacteria can undergo a pleomorphic change to accommodate the digestive needs of the new food. By the time a child is two years old, there may be as many as 400 variations of bacteria in the gastrointestinal tract, and the child is ready for the basic challenges of digestion. By a supercoordinated effort, his baby teeth have all erupted and are ready to make their important contribution to the process of food digestion. From here on, let's refer to the gastrointestinal tract as the "G.I. tract."

Mercury the Marauder

When mercury is placed in the mouth in the form of silver mercury fillings (as often occurs by age two years), both mechanical and chemical conditions stimulate the release of mercury out of the fillings into the mouth. When the mechanical condition is chewing, mercury readily mixes with the foods and is swallowed with the food. In the stomach and G.I. tract, mercury comes in contact with the "friendly" bacteria. Not being too friendly itself, mercury may kill the bacteria. If the bacteria are a bit more hardy, they may undergo another alteration (pleomorphic change) such that they are more resistant to mercury. Altered intestinal bacteria almost digest your food properly, but not quite. The resultant *almost* properly digested foods are absorbed into the bloodstream; while almost the right shape and form, they do not fool the immune system. Your immune system is especially programmed to attack anything that does not look right. In these cases, the immune system's attack on almost properly digested proteins can produce a reaction referred to as an allergic reaction. Many people report an improvement in their allergies after amalgam removal. Perhaps the resultant increase in properly digested protein and decrease of altered protein after mercury removal is part of the reason.

Altered bacteria also encourage the rotting of proteins called putrefaction. Putrefaction of proteins results in the production of more toxins that interfere with the actual absorptive mechanism from the intestinal lining. As a result of these injuries, the selective absorption of the tract is improper, allowing a seepage of partially processed foods to go through the lining into the body itself. The lymphatic drainage system picks up these weird molecules and channels them into the blood vessels. "Leaky gut syndrome" is one of the labels applied to this situation.

When incompletely digested food particles are allowed access to the bloodstream, immune surveillance mechanisms are triggered. Your immune system is trained to attack anything that does not look right, or "self," and incompletely digested food particles really do not "look right." The immune system sees these particles as foreign substances called antigens, and launches an attack against them, which is one of the primary ways in which food allergies are developed. In this way, mercury can turn every meal into an immune challenge instead of the nutritional boost it is supposed to be.

Another way in which bacteria can create a problem is to add a piece of DNA from a dead bacterium onto the end of its own DNA. This little addition is called a plasmid. A bacterium with a plasmid is resistant to mercury and can live in its presence, where other, unmodified bacteria might die.

Plasmid formation results in another important effect. Many plasmid-reinforced bacteria simultaneously become resistant to certain antibiotics. Tetracycline is one of the most common antibiotics to demonstrate this resistance, but it can happen to many other antibiotics as well.

It is possible that the presence of mercury in the mouth, and subsequently in the G.I. tract, is one of the major factors in the increase in antibiotic resistance. Resistance is emerging so rapidly now that drug companies are producing new antibiotic variations every month or two in an attempt to stay ahead of these wily, resistant bacterial strains.

Candidly Speaking

Another important interrelationship between mercury and G.I. bacteria deserves specific mention. *Candida albicans* is a yeast that is normally found in the G.I. tract, but only in limited numbers. In people without oral heavy-metal contamination, the friendly bacteria in the G.I. tract have specific assignments. One of the assignments is for certain bacteria to exercise population control over candida. If the candida count gets too high, then the normal bacteria assigned to that task are supposed to kill off the excess candida. When mercury enters the G.I. environment, sometimes these controlling bacteria are killed or distorted and receive a different job description, leaving candida free to multiply undisturbed.

Candida has strange eating habits. Much of its energy needs can be met by converting methylmercury into inorganic mercury. The energy absorbed sustains its daily needs. In a nicely reciprocal arrangement, some of the G.I. bacteria can then take the inorganic mercury produced by the candida and reconvert it into methylmercury. Then the candida converts it into inorganic mercury, and we have a system similar to perpetual motion. As long as there is at least one mercury filling in the mouth, this system can continue indefinitely. This is why taking drugs to kill candida is effective only while taking them. As soon the drugs are stopped, the candida numbers increase again and the symptoms associated with candida overgrowth return.

Gut Responses

Another reaction of mercury in the gut can be diarrhea. Although potentially disruptive to one's lifestyle, diarrhea is an effective response by the body to rid the G.I. tract of harmful or toxic substances that may have been ingested. Whenever the toxin is chronically administered, as with amalgam fillings and the regular eating of mercury-laden seafood, diarrhea can become a chronic problem.

From the patients that we saw at Huggins Diagnostic Center, it was apparent that after a certain period of time the pattern of chronic diarrhea would often cycle to a pattern of alternating diarrhea and constipation, and eventually settle into chronic constipation. Although there is a wide range in the length of time this takes to occur, it appears to average about eight years from the time the body begins to fight the presence of mercury seriously with the onset of diarrhea until the appearance of total chronic constipation.

The phase of chronic constipation leads to another G.I.-related issue. Parasites. Parasitic infections cause the sick patient to become even sicker. Not only do parasites rob these patients of essential nutrients, but they supply their own toxic by-products as well.

Where do the parasites come from? Fruits, vegetables, and lovable pets can be laden with parasites that can provide a constant bombardment to our system. Normally our immune system can control these exposures, but along with constipation comes the reduced ability of the immune system to remove parasites.

Chemical removal of parasites is difficult and rarely permanently effective if the initial reason for the infestation is not eliminated. Making the living environment uninviting for the parasites through promoting toxin-free, healthy bodies and immune systems is the only real long-term answer to their control.

Immune Protection

After mercury filling removal, the immune system has a chance to recover. It then develops a severe resentment toward any reintroduction of mercury into the body and builds a protective early-warning system. The development of this immune protective system typically requires three to six months of a relatively mercury-free existence. This is known as a secondary immune response.

This response is a protective response, but it certainly does not feel like protection. After recovery, should you get a new mercury exposure, usually from eating some kind of fresh- or saltwater fish, your immune system may decide to purge your body of the mercury exposure by giving you a serious case of diarrhea for a day or two. Purpose? To rapidly get rid of the villain mercury. Try to remember that this is a "protective" response. You may think that your body is trying to punish you, but in actuality, it is trying to save you from mercury exposure. Many times when people have a G.I. reaction to what they consider exposure to "bad" seafood, it may well be a reaction to an unusually high level of methylmercury in the seafood.

Toxic Roots

In many of our patients, we noted that, historically, they didn't have significant digestive problems until after one or more root canals were performed. Only recently have we found out what the connection is between mercury, root canals, and digestive problems. The common denominator appears to be toxic immune damage, whether from a heavy metal like mercury, or from a bacterial toxin, as from a root canal treated tooth. A similar problem can occur in people who have periodontal (gum) disease, because some of the same toxins are produced in diseased gums.

From 1995 through 1997, we have studied the toxins that are often found in the periodontal ligament surrounding the root canal tooth. (For a detailed explanation, see chapter 11, on root canals.) These toxins are formed within the root structure of the tooth itself, regardless of what is used to fill the root canal. Once formed, these toxins migrate to the outside of the root to the interphase between bone and tooth. When one bites down, as during chewing, a few molecules of the toxins are forced up the root surface into the mouth. From the mouth, toxins are mixed with saliva and foods and swallowed into the stomach and intestinal tract. These toxins are unaffected by the acids and enzymes in the stomach.

By performing gel electrophoresis, these toxins can be separated and put into dilute solutions (in the part per billion range) of known amounts of normal enzymes. One can then determine just how toxic the root canal exudates are. So far there is nothing known in biochemistry or toxicology that is quite as toxic per volume as these root canal-generated toxins. The degree of toxicity created by root canal bacteria is literally close to the molecular level.

It takes microminute amounts of this substance (called Acute Dentally Associated toxins by the University of Kentucky) only a minute or two to inactivate many of the body's most critical enzymes.

One of the enzymes tested was a glycolytic enzyme. Glycolytic enzymes are critical for the breakdown of glucose (thus the glyco portion of its name), which is the critical energy substance for life in all cells. Now let's go to the site of action to see specifically how these toxins alter normal metabolism.

During normal digestion, foods are broken down in the mouth and stomach and prepared for the more involved phase of digestion that takes place in the intestines.

The first layer of the intestine in contact with the food is called the epithelium. These epithelial cells contain glycolytic enzymes that are critical in the production of trypsin, chymotrypsin, and pepsin, which are primary digestive enzymes. After these digestive enzymes are manufactured, they are released from the epithelial cells into the digestive tract. Enzyme action on the food allows its breakdown into basic nutrient components that can then be absorbed into the bloodstream through other cells in the small intestine.

As toxins from root canal teeth are released into the saliva, they mix with other components of the saliva, one of which will be mercury if there are any silver mercury amalgam fillings implanted in the teeth. In addition to the newly discovered toxins, several other toxic chemicals are produced simultaneously in the periodontal ligament space. Among these are hydrogen sulfide and methyl mercaptan. As this team of chemicals is exposed to mercury, an immediate reaction occurs between them and a new "dual" toxin is formed that can easily enter the epithelial cells of the intestinal tract. As they enter the epithelial cell, the glycolytic enzymes are promptly killed, substantially inhibiting the production of trypsin, chymotrypsin, and pepsin that are necessary for complete digestion. The inhibition of this enzyme production is another reason for the development of chronic constipation.

Chronic constipation can easily lead to chronic laxative abuse. Laxatives can have a number of effects. In addition to altering the fluid balance of the G.I. tract, they cause the epithelial cells to sluff off the intestinal wall in order to move the digesting food mass along. This results in the loss of those important enzyme-producing cells. The combination of all of this damage to the intestinal tract together with the resultant loss of raw materials for proper metabolism sets the stage for developing a wide range of G.I. diseases, including cancer.

A Good Start

The complexity of this entire process of digestion glosses over what is probably the most significant factor to good digestion (and its influence on good health in general): Thorough chewing.

Root canal and mercury toxicity is not required to impair the digestion of hastily gulped food. The entire sequence of events leading to the leaky gut syndrome and chronic immune system stress and multiple food allergies does not require the contribution of mercury toxicity. Merely allowing chunks of food to reach the stomach in an unprepared state will easily facilitate the same outcome.

Chunks of food can only rot in your body. They cannot be properly digested. It is true that a snake has the digestive power to completely digest a rat swallowed whole without chewing, but a human being's digestive enzymes must have food preprocessed into a semiliquid form by thorough chewing. Anything less will diminish a diet's nutritive benefit and simultaneously increase the toxic effects of that poorly digested food.

So, remember to chew. It doesn't cost anything, and it may be singularly more beneficial to your general health than any one thing that you can do. Regardless of your level of toxicity, nutrition (in which proper diet is properly prepared for digestion) is your best front-line defense. And remember that chewing is the primary factor in helping you reach that goal.

Know the Price

So you chew well, but you still have root canals and amalgams. What do you do? The easy answer is to remove any source of chronic toxicity. But what if your root canal tooth is not producing measurable toxins? Dr. Weston Price's research indicates that all root canal teeth can eventually become toxic. Onset is related to when your defenses are compromised enough to allow a disease to become established. An easy test to measure the toxicity of a root canal tooth without extracting it has not yet been refined. Such testing procedures are under development, and hopefully may be available soon, but it is not here yet; so let's look at the options.

We know that mercury can cause digestive problems by itself. We know that the additional presence of root canals or other nonvital teeth increases the potential for developing more digestive problems. We know that not 100% of the root canals are instrumental in developing digestive problems. Maybe you can relate the onset of digestive problems to a period of time around six months prior to your first needing a root canal. This would make it easy. Now that you are informed of the potential with mercury and with root canals, you may choose whatever path makes you comfortable. You know your options.

Reference for this Chapter

Price, W. A. 1923. *Dental Infections, Oral and Systemic,* vol. 1. Cleveland: Penton Publishing Co.

5

Leukemia: Listening Instead of Lecturing

I (HH) got a personal introduction to leukemia and my first exposure to dental toxicity jointly in 1973 when I met Dr. Olympio Pinto. I was lecturing to an international group on the use of blood chemistry interpretation to control dental decay and gum disease, and had mentioned one gum condition that did not respond despite the fact that all the chemistries said it should have. Pinto came up to me after the program and told me that this particular gum condition was not responding because mercury was coming out of the silver mercury fillings into the gums of those patients. I argued the "party line" that mercury was tightly bound within the amalgam, and therefore it was inert and completely harmless. After some argument about whether or not mercury could, in fact, come out of the filling, I began to listen. That was my first real learning experience. Learning to repeat what others have told you is one thing, but learning to think and challenge the old guard was an entirely new experience. New to me, not to Olympio.

Olympio told me of a six-year-old child that was referred to his dentist father in the 1920s. The child had leukemia, and her only complaint was that her gums hurt. The elder Dr. Pinto was asked to clean the child's teeth to see if that would help her discomfort. Pinto felt that leukemia was a reaction to mercury and proceeded to remove her silver mercury amalgam fillings. The child experienced a remarkable spontaneous remission the next day.

"Wait a minute," I interrupted, "we were talking about gum disease. Leukemia is cancer. This is a serious accusation."

"Just listen to the rest of the story if you think that is challenging," Olympio responded. The elder Pinto had explained to the doctors what he had done. They scoffed at him and told him that dental mercury had nothing to do with leukemia. Leukemia was a medical disease. Rather than argue the point, Pinto replaced the amalgam fillings. Leukemia returned. Having made his point, he then removed the fillings a second time and the child lived leukemia free.

Hearing of this event impacted me in a way I had never experienced before. Pinto the younger then said, "Look, you know how to interpret chemistry changes. Go home, place mercury fillings, remove them, monitor the blood changes, and decide for yourself whether or not mercury in fillings affects people's health adversely." Within three weeks, I had given away my amalgam filling equipment along with my entire stock of mercury.

Mechanisms

Leukemia is a disease of the bone marrow in which white blood cells are produced in tremendous excesses. White blood cells normally respond to toxic challenges that have entered the body through the mouth, nose, a break in the skin, or otherwise have accessed the inner body, where they do not belong. The objective of these immune cells is to destroy the invading challenge by eating it (phagocytosis) or inactivating it through creating destructive enzymes. If the normal standby population of cells is not enough, more cells can be produced rapidly. The type of leukemia that results in an overproduction of white cells may be an overzealous immune response to a toxic challenge—such as mercury from dental amalgams.

Leukemia may also take the form of an exhausted immune response. In these cases, the white blood cells are low. They may drop to 2,000 cells per cubic millimeter or less. The entire mechanism of the disease may be different from the elevated form of leukemia. Minor infections will often become overwhelming in these patients, for they do not have enough white cells to fight effectively even against minor challenges.

An unchallenged, "normal" white cell count will run between five and ten thousand cells per cubic milliliter. In the overproduction forms of leukemias, cellular counts can reach over 200,000 cells in their active stages.

Two of the accepted medical treatments are irradiation and chemotherapy, in which it is hoped that the malignant runaway cells are eliminated faster than normal cells. This goal does not always occur in reality.

Additional Factors Influencing Leukemia

Genetics and environmental factors are both influential in the development of leukemia. Identical twins will both develop leukemia 40 times more often than nontwin brothers and sisters. Environmentally, chromosomal alterations as created by exposures to radiation have been implicated in its onset. Chromosomal alterations resulting in leukemia are not always the same. Sometimes the alterations produce an increased number of chromosomes (hyperdiploid), sometimes a decreased number (hypodiploid), sometimes an exchange of parts of chromosomes (translocation). The identical chromosomes are not always affected either, although numbers 9 and 22 are the most common.

DNA lesions produced by mercury are different from lesions created by other agents. Most damage to the DNA is in the form of breaks in the intertwined strands (called single strand breaks) and they are readily repaired by (reductase) enzymes. In the case of mercury-caused breakage, the breaks are not readily repaired. DNA-DNA crosslinks, or binding of two DNAs together, is another malignant form of chromosomal damage that is created by mercury. It could be considered a hyperdiploid form of leukemia.

Uncontested Leakage of Mercury from Amalgam

It is well documented that mercury continually seeps out of the silver-mercury amalgam filling. As early as 1979, Gay and others reported that amalgam fillings at rest emitted mercury vapor levels of 2.8 micrograms per cubic meter of air. With stimulation from chewing gum, that level rose to as high as 49 micrograms. That stimulated level of mercury vapor vastly exceeded the "safe" exposure level of 10 micrograms established in many European countries. Various levels, ranging from 25 to 50 micrograms, are established as safe in the United States. In a political (non-scientific) gesture to make dentists feel comfortable placing mercury, the ADA recognizes 500 micrograms as safe. Svare, repeating Gay's work in 1981, recorded values up to 87.5 micrograms after chewing gum. This 15,600 percent increase was astronomically higher than the values found before chewing gum.

Even higher levels could be anticipated with hot foods or foods with acidic properties. Vinegar-and-oil salad dressing is wonderful for digestion, but the vinegar can release substantial amounts of mercury from amalgam fillings into the foods.

It is also known that mercury can cause damage to the chromosomes within a cell. Mercury has effects similar to those created by X-ray exposure, like being able to produce oxygen radicals in cells and depleting cellular reduced glutathione levels; thus the DNA must be considered a target site of mercury's toxic action.

Actions and Reactions

At that initial meeting with Dr. Pinto, he had told me to monitor white blood cells because they were quite responsive to the presence or absence of mercury. Yes, they had changed. So did some of the blood chemistries. Those changes, along with changes in the people themselves, played a big role in my decision to stop placing amalgams.

After many years of observing changes in white blood cells, I published an article listing a few of the observations I had made.

Over the years, I had noted that amalgam removal was followed by drops in the high levels of white blood cells. It also encouraged increases in the low levels of white cells. This article summarized some of those changes.

Not mentioned in the article, but observed nonetheless, was the fact that even the levels from 6,000 to 10,000 had a tendency to seek the area between 5,000 and 6,000. There was sort of an optimum level for the unchallenged immune system that was adequate for standby, but not overtaxing for the immune system. It looked like the optimum level was 5,000 to 6,000, and in some people, even the presence of one or two amalgams would increase the white cell level to 7,000 or 8,000. Then a thought occurred to me. Is it possible that leukemia is a valiant attempt on the part of a super-healthy immune system to rid the body of a challenge that the system considers extremely bad? Compromised immune systems cannot launch more than a moderate attack against invaders, but what about the really healthy system? Would it produce legions of white cell fighters? In the process of failure after failure to rid the body of the challenge, does something go awry and get stuck in the overproduction mode? Just like in other cancers?

Amazing Anecdotes or Natural Reactions?

A number of specific cases support this suggestion. With this amalgam-leukemia connection in mind, we began to remove amalgams and other toxic materials from people with leukemia. The case reports are here for you to evaluate. First, there is the original Pinto case. If you will glance at the graph, you will notice that there is one patient who was undergoing chemotherapy, and still had a count of 235,000. He had only a few amalgams, and all were removed in one day. (I wouldn't do it that way today.) In two days—being a doctor and having made the decision to take himself off chemotherapy—his white cell count dropped to 176,000, a drop of 59,000.

Another striking case dropped from 73,700 to 12,700, a 61,000-count drop in one week following amalgam removal. Even if changes this striking do not occur every time, the fact that they do occur suggests strongly that there is some significant cause-and-effect relationship between mercury amalgam fillings and the white blood cell count. Referring again to the graph, it seems to be the

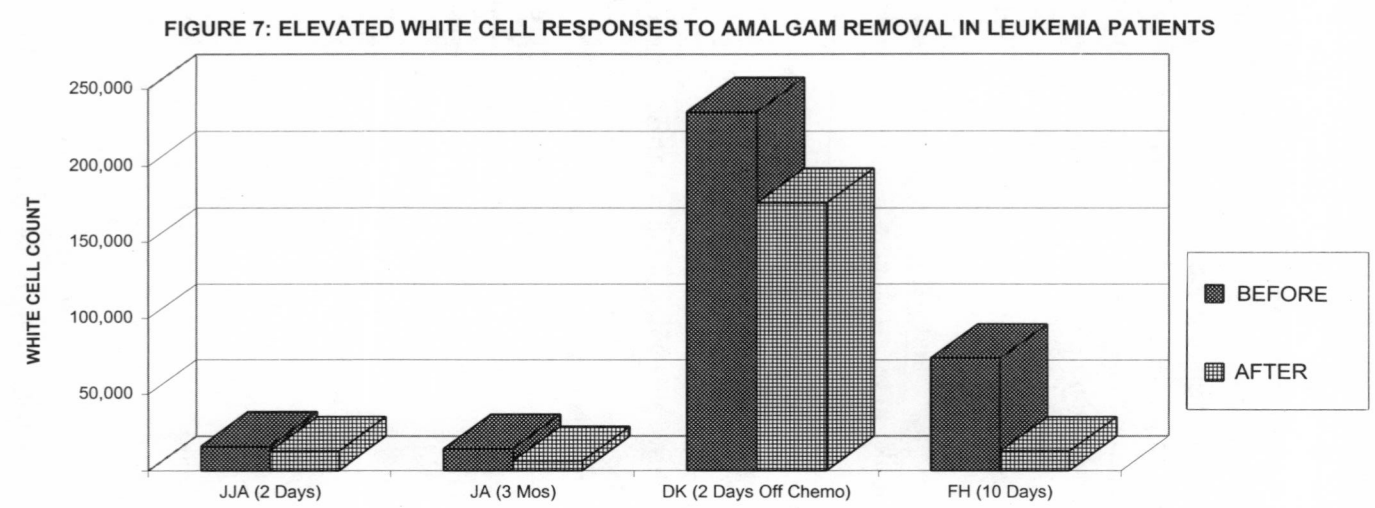

FIGURE 7: ELEVATED WHITE CELL RESPONSES TO AMALGAM REMOVAL IN LEUKEMIA PATIENTS

rule, not the exception, for amalgam removal to lower elevated white cell counts.

A five-year-old girl was in my office while her older sister was being treated. Her father mentioned that she had recently lost over twenty pounds. That's a lot of weight for a five-year-old to lose. Her energy level was notably lower than usual, but the family thought that was due to the frequent trips the father had to take because of his position. Out of curiosity I drew her blood and tested it. Her white cell count was more than 16,000. She had two amalgam fillings that were removed the same day we noted the elevated count. The very next day her count had dropped over 10,000 to a more healthy 6,000.

Clinicians who deal with white cell elevations as a response to infection do not typically see such dramatic shifts, for infections generally resolve gradually rather than abruptly. It has become obvious that when a toxic challenge is removed abruptly, an equally abrupt shift in white cell count can be anticipated.

A young lady in her mid-twenties came to our office just prior to going to Seattle for a bone marrow transplant. Although the removal of her dental toxicity was performed only a few weeks before the bone marrow transplant, the procedure appeared to benefit her significantly. Her doctors reported that she recovered faster than anyone they had ever treated.

One dentist with over twenty years of mercury exposure in his dental office was helping his parents by cleaning out the bottom of their wheat storage bin. He noticed a peculiar sight—one that should have triggered some alarm. Several rats were crawling around slowly, appearing to have near paralysis of their hind legs. Following this, his shovel splashed into a silvery liquid at the bottom of the bin. Mercury. His father explained that pouring several pounds of mercury in the bottom of the bin was standard procedure. It reduced the rat population.

Within a few days, the dentist was diagnosed with leukemia. Because his white cell count was around 80,000, immediate chemotherapy was recommended. He declined chemotherapy, having seen the consequences in more than one person, and opted for amalgam removal instead. We removed his amalgams, did the other procedures found necessary to help the mercury-toxic patient, and the count came down to 20,000, but would drop no further. I thought a mild protocol of chemotherapy might be a useful adjunct, but he refused. He declined and never went back to the twelve-hour working days of his earlier practice. He coped with his condition very well and enjoyed a much less hectic (and less toxic) lifestyle.

These chemistries and cases are a sampling of what leads me to think that you need to be informed of the potentials of mercury exposure—especially if your genetics are predisposed to leukemia. Surely not all cases of leukemia are initiated in the dental office, yet I still remember that amalgam was initiated commercially in 1832, and leukemia was first described in 1845.

Leukemia presents not just a medical challenge, but a political one as well. Take the following case as an example and determine what you would do if faced with the same situation. An eight-year-old boy had two amalgams placed on a Friday. He became fussy on Saturday and complained that his gums hurt. By Sunday the child was diagnosed with leukemia. Grandmother had read my book *It's All in Your Head* and suggested to the doctors that they consider having the amalgams removed. Immediately the parents' and grandparents' "rights to free medical choice" were removed and the child was made a ward of the state. The child was started on six different kinds of chemotherapy.

The grandmother called me to seek information. If leukemia started that quickly after amalgam placement, what would be the harm in removing the two amalgams? Sounded okay to me. The doctors had many reasons why that should not be done. After six weeks, the grandmother prevailed and the doctors allowed the fillings to be removed. Although the white cells recovered by the next day, the doctors refused to inform the parents for seven days. Even so, they refused to consider a relationship between amalgam removal and the disappearance of the leukemia. They continued to scoff at the family any time the subject was breached.

Even though the white cells were okay, the doctors elected to give him another round of chemotherapy just to be on the safe side. With no real disease present, he responded poorly and his spleen expanded, so they removed his spleen. He is now off chemotherapy and has experienced a marvelous case of "spontaneous remission."

Just Consider It!

Even though there are four different general classifications of leukemia, we have not noted a particular difference between them in response to dental revision. This information is not meant to assert that every case of leukemia has a dental component, but the possibility of such a critical connection should never be overlooked in the primary evaluation of any case of leukemia.

If you have been faced with a similar situation relative to the placement of fillings (or root canals or children's pulp caps for that matter) and the onset of leukemia, please check our Web site at www.hugnet.com.

References for this Chapter

Cantoni, O., M. Costa. 1983. Correlations of DNA strand breaks and their repair with cell survival following acute exposure to mercury (II) and X-rays. *Molecular Pharmocology* 24:84-89.

Cantoni, O., et al. 1983. Possible involvement of superoxide free radicals in the $HgCl_2$ induced DNA damage in CHO cells. *Fed. Proc.* 42:1135.

Cantoni, O., et al. 1982. Similarity in the acute cytotoxic response to mammalian cells to mercury (II) and X-rays. DNA damage and glutathione depletion. *Biochemical and Biophysical Research Communications* 108:614.

Gay, D. D., R. C. Cox, J. W. Reinhard. 1982. Chewing releases mercury from fillings. *Lancet*.

Huggins, H. A. 1989. Proposed role of dental amalgam toxicity in leukemia and hematopoietic dyscrasias. *International Journal of Biosocial and Medical Research* 11:84-93.

Schimpff, S. C., V. M. Young, W. H. Greene. 1972. Origin of infections in acute nonlymphocytic leukemia. *Annals of International Medicine* 77:707-714.

Svare, C. W., et al. September 1981. The effect of dental amalgams on mercury levels in expired air. *Journal of Dental Research* 60(9): 1668-71.

6

Cholesterol and Dentistry: Strange Bedfellows

Protector or Provoker?

Following the lead of one of my early mentors, Melvin E. Page, D.D.S., I (HH) have been balancing body chemistries, including cholesterol levels, through nutrition and supplementation for three decades. Cholesterol has always warranted special attention because of its important role in the control of dental decay and gum disease. As a result of balancing cholesterol levels for many years, I certainly suspected that I had a reasonable awareness of the most important variables that affected cholesterol. The 1996 Coors Study changed that opinion. The Coors Study pointed out that amalgam had a direct and adverse effect on cholesterol levels. There is no substitute for being there.

No other laboratory test captures the attention of either the medical community or the lay public more than the *serum cholesterol level*. The primary reason for this is the solidly established connection between coronary heart disease and elevated cholesterol levels. Many primary prevention clinical trials, such as those reported by F. T. Hatch and P. K. Reissell, have demonstrated that various cholesterol-lowering measures can lower the incidence of heart disease. The obvious conclusion is that elevated cholesterol is undesirable. Reaching this conclusion is not as straightforward as it may seem at first. A definite correlation between two things does not always constitute the presence of a cause-and-effect relationship.

Over the past two decades, a new cholesterol concern has been raised. It is now recognized that there are even *greater* concerns about the negative health impacts of *low* serum cholesterol levels. The effects of the low levels may be even more important, even though they have not received the same media attention as high cholesterol.

Death from any cause is undesirable, whether it comes from heart disease or cancer. Given the choice, most people would choose death from a heart attack over death from cancer. Most of the information you are about to read remains largely unknown even though it has been published in respectable medical journals. Focusing on low cholesterol is not easy in a world medical community that is still conditioned to think that lower cholesterol levels are associated with better health.

Recent research indicated that the death rate due to heart disease in males aged forty-five to fifty-four was 62 per 100,000 population. This cardiac death rate is significantly reduced when the cholesterol levels are reduced below 200 milligrams percent (mg%), or 200 milligrams of cholesterol per 100 milliliters of blood serum. The incidence of cardiac death remained lowered with further reduction of the cholesterol levels below 160 mg%, but the overall *rate of death* nearly *doubled*. It increased to 107 deaths per 100,000 men. The increased deaths were due to cancer, suicide, violent deaths, and cerebral hemorrhage.

The puzzle of why cholesterol-lowering trials fail to lower total mortality from all causes can be explained when one considers the possibility that a clinically significant amount of mercury is chronically released from amalgam fillings. Low-grade mercury poisoning (micromercurialism) can have many symptoms, but none are more prominent than irritability, depression, and emotional instability.

Increased deaths from suicide and violence when cholesterol levels get too low may represent an aggravation of low-grade mercury toxicity no longer being effectively neutralized by the lower cholesterol levels. Depression and irritability taken to their limits could manifest themselves as suicide and violence. If cholesterol protects against the harmful effects of mercury, then less protection could be expected to result in a greater incidence of cancer. Mercury is known to target DNA, which can lead to cancer-producing mutations.

Cholesterol serves as a major protector in normal metabolism, primarily through its inactivation of toxic substances. This includes mercury and other heavy metals. Cholesterol has many other little-emphasized functions. They include positive effects on the fluidity of cell membranes, membrane permeability, transmembrane exchange, and neuronal signal transmission. Cholesterol provides the major framework on which the five major classes of steroid hormones are manufactured. Fat-soluble vitamins, antioxidants, drugs, and toxins all use cholesterol in a transport capacity. The ability to neutralize a wide variety of toxins is only one of a wide variety of tasks that cholesterol performs.

A review of the medical literature reveals that cholesterol has been identified as an inactivator of multiple bacterial toxins in animals. Further, high cholesterol levels appear to be indicators of toxic exposures. Cholesterol levels rise in people with occupational exposure to pesticides. A high cholesterol level appears to indicate a healthy response of a body trying to cope with a high toxin load that cannot be eliminated. If the body becomes ill, it may be because of the high unneutralized toxin load present, and *not* because of the high cholesterol level attempting to achieve the neutralization.

Contrasting sharply with the low-fat craze that has seized the population, we have found that adding substantial amounts of good fats to the diet improves the blood chemistry and clinical appearances of patients. Patients completing dental revision would sometimes show drops of cholesterol of 50 mg% or more within a week. Their diet included two eggs and a stick of butter a day. Most people were certain their cholesterol levels would shoot off the chart. This simply did not happen. The cholesterol levels paralleled the degree of toxic challenge present at the time the blood was drawn. Lower levels of cholesterol tended to come up after dental revision as reliably as the higher levels would drop. In a small percentage of patients, it appeared that mercury could actually interfere with the body's production of cholesterol. Low cholesterol levels would often correlate with poorer health because sicker patients tended to have less protection against toxicity.

Coors and Cholesterol

The Coors Study provided us with information about the effects of amalgam removal alone on cholesterol levels. No dietary changes were advised, and no cholesterol-lowering drugs were involved. Data from twenty-eight people was obtained. Amalgam was the only dental material in the mouth. No braces, crowns, root canals, or other immune-altering materials were present. After initial blood testing, the amalgams were removed and replaced with a composite (plastic material) that had been tested against the blood to make sure it was compatible with the immune system. The next blood test followed a minimum of eight days later. There was a striking trend in the cholesterol levels in all subjects. (Please see graph.) Most high cholesterol levels came down, and most low cholesterol levels came up. Of the 74% of subjects showing decreases, drops ranged from just a few mg% to over 40 mg%. Remember that this was with amalgam removal alone. When total dental revision is performed, we have consistently seen responses that are even more dramatic. This indicates that the whole multidisciplined program that we advocate does an even better job. Until the Coors Study was done, we had no idea of how a big an effect amalgam removal alone had on cholesterol levels.

Other published data showed a U-shaped curve, where cancer and violent deaths were found associated with low cholesterol levels and heart disease deaths were found associated with high cholesterol levels. The bottom of the "U," where few deaths of either variety were noted, mathematically settled on a cholesterol level of 221 mg%. Assembled from over 9,000 people, this data warrants a reasonable amount of credibility. Interestingly enough, in 1968 Dr. Page noted that after fifty years of study and thousands of patients, he had found the "optimum" cholesterol level to be 222 mg%.

The influence of amalgam on cholesterol levels is something that everyone should know, especially when there is a family history of heart disease, cancer, or any other disease for which toxicity can be a causative or significantly contributing factor. As always, you have the right to be informed.

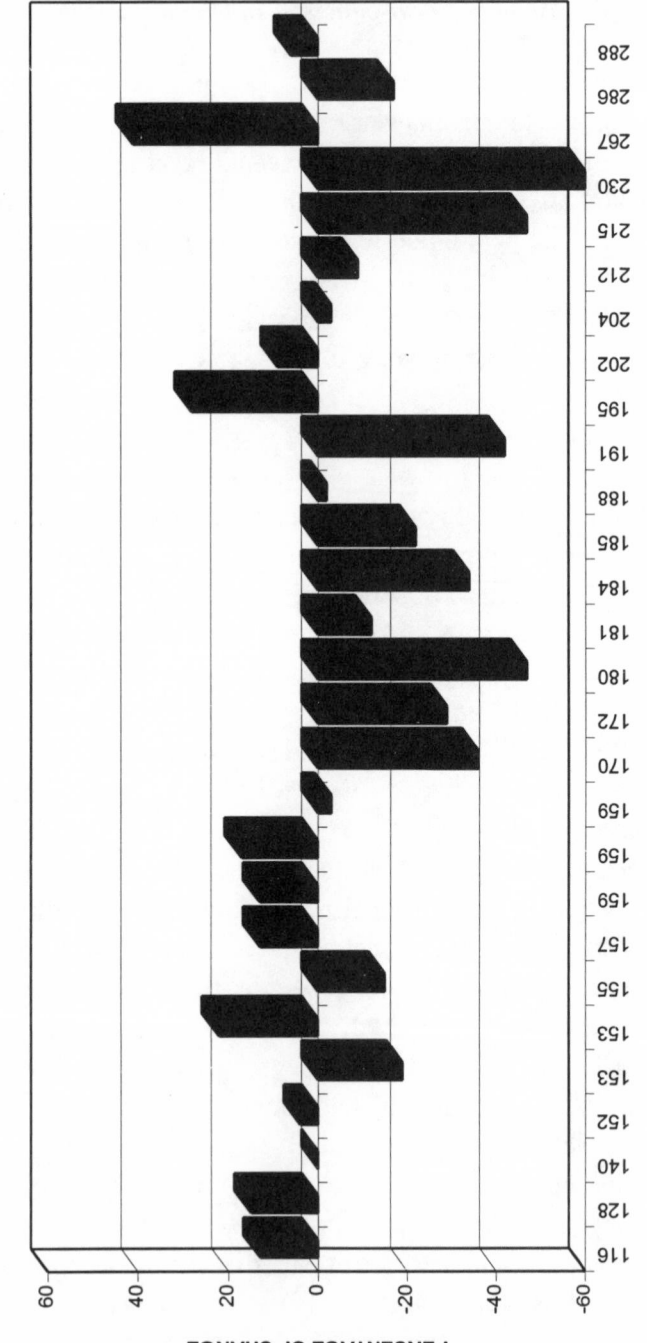

FIGURE 8: CHANGES IN CHOLESTEROL VALUES AFTER AMALGAM REMOVAL

References for this Chapter

Alouf, J. E. September-December 1981. [Les toxines cytolytiques bacteriennes thiol-dependantes: streptolysine O et toxines apparentees.] Thiol-dependent cytolytic bacterial toxins: streptolysin O and prominent toxins. *Archives de l'Institute Pasteur de Tunis* 58(3):355-73.

Bloomer A. W., S. I. Nash, H. A. Price, R. L. Welch. December 1977. A study of pesticide residues in Michigan's general population. 1968-70. *Pestic Monit J* 11(3):111-5.

Fielding, D. J., et al. 1982. Cholesterol transport between cells and body fluids. *Medical Clinics of North America* 66:363-373.

Hatch F. T., et al. 1966. A study of coronary heart disease in young men: Characteristics and metabolic studies of patients and comparison with age matched healthy controls. *Circulation* 33:679-703.

Jacobs D., et al. 1992. Report of the conference on low blood cholesterol: Mortality associations. *Circulation* 86 (3):1047.

Kaplan, J. R., S. B. Manuck. 1990. The effects of fat and cholesterol on aggressive behavior in monkeys. *Psychosomatic Medicine* 52: 226-7.

Page, Melvin, H. Leon Abrams, Jr. 1971. *Health Versus Disease* 2nd ed. Newport Beach, Calif.: The Page Foundation.

Pekkanen, J., et al. 1989. Serum cholesterol and risk of accidental or violent death in a 25 year follow-up. *Archives of Internal Medicine* 49:1589-91.

Schatzhin, A., R. N. Hoover, et al. 1990. Serum cholesterol levels and cancer in the NHANES Epidemiologic Followup Study. *Lancet* 2:298-301.

Virkkunen, M., H. Penttinen. 1984. Serum cholesterol in aggressive conduct disorder, a preliminary study. *Biological Psychiatry* 19:435-439.

7

The Results of
Interference with Hormones

Hormones are powerful chemicals in our bodies. Only a few micrograms will elicit a response within us. The most obvious is probably adrenalin. When life-threatening danger poses a challenge, we can feel the adrenalin rush within a second or two. Hormones are very influential compared to their weight. I (HH) have heard it stated that the amount of estrogen manufactured per lifetime is equal to the weight of a postage stamp.

Hormones that are most often affected by mercury are thyroid, insulin, estrogen, testosterone, both anterior and posterior pituitary, and adrenalin.

Many hormones have activators. Thyroid, for example, requires iodine to be complete. If iodine cannot connect with thyroid, then the hormone, for practical purposes, is inactivated. This is the vulnerable spot often attacked by mercury. Almost all hormones have binding sights capable of connecting to metabolic cofactors, but mercury can bind here, too. In fact, mercury frequently has a stronger affinity for those binding sites than the normal activators. When mercury binds, the original intent of the hormone is altered, and, even though the hormone is present in the bloodstream, it may not be able to act as it is supposed to.

Thyroid

Let's talk about hormones one at a time regarding their dental relationships. Thyroid is a good place to start. Thyroid actually has four binding sites for iodine. Should mercury attach to one of these sites, the hormone activity will be altered.

Dr. D. C. Jarvis, a medical doctor on the East Coast, founded a metabolic study club in the early 1900s that ran for almost fifty years. There were sixty medical doctors and two dentists as members for most of its existence. A dentist from Florida named Dr. Melvin Page was the secretary. Through Page, I learned about the function of endocrine glands and their relation to both medical and dental health. The two seem to be closely intertwined.

Dental decay

Thyroid is one of the important glands influencing dental decay. There is a fluid flow from the pulp chamber, through the dentin, through the enamel and into the mouth in people who have no dental decay. Thyroid offers part of the endocrine function that controls the direction of this fluid flow. Low thyroid hormone production allows this fluid flow to run in the opposite direction—from the mouth, into the enamel, dentin, and pulp chamber. This fluid brings bacteria and debris from the mouth with it, leading to dental decay. Jarvis and his group noted that decay was associated with a blood serum phosphorus level of less than 3.5 milligrams percent. In fact the group found that when the teeth were susceptible to decay, the whole body was susceptible to degenerative disease.

Which one? Whichever was involved with your genetic weak link. They found that dispensing small amounts of thyroid to hypothyroid patients who had dental decay drastically reduced the decay rate. Records I saw indicated that some people with rampant decay went over ten years without a new cavity. So hormones are an integral part of susceptibility to dental decay.

Body temperature

Thyroid is involved with maintenance of proper body temperature. The optimum body temperature is 98.6 degrees Fahrenheit. We have noted that most mercury toxic patients have lower than optimum body temperatures. The most toxic patients may have readings as low as 96.2. When the amalgam fillings are removed, there is a trend for the temperature to approach 98.6. I have personally seen body temperature move from 96.5 to 98.4 within twenty-four hours of removing all of the amalgams. In that case, there were only six small amalgams, and they were all removed at one appointment. I would not do it that way today, but this was twenty years ago, before we knew the protocol that we know today.

It is possible that the high-copper amalgams have even more influence on body temperature than the older, conventional amalgam. Mercury comes out of the high-copper amalgam fillings 50 times faster, so there is foundation for the suspicion. Of practical interest, I read in one of the journals a year or so ago that the medical profession is considering lowering the normal body temperature level of 98.6 because so many people have lower temperatures. My suggestion is to leave the optimum body temperature where it is, and get rid of the mercury.

Emotions and the thyroid

Emotions are complex, and yes, they are influenced by what happens to us. Perhaps a bigger influence yet is how hormonal levels can intertwine with our external environmental influences. We all know really negative people who are unhappy with everything that happens, and others that are happy regardless of what "goes wrong." You know, the "so let's make lemonade" type. A large portion of this attitude adjustment is related to thyroid levels.

It is not unusual to have a patient's feeling of well being increase within a day or two of having fillings replaced . . . when the proper protocol is used. If the protocol is violated, then the opposite reaction may result. Can you measure feelings of well being? Not that I know about, but the patients surely experience it.

Let's not forget unexplained depression. Note the word *unexplained*. It is critical in the diagnosis of mercury toxicity. If someone just ran into your brand-new car, okay, depression can be a natural outgrowth. But when it happens after winning the lottery, hey, wait a minute, something else is going on. In a study of symptoms we collected on 1,320 people, depression was the winner. It occurred 73% of the time. Unexplained anxiety was close to it at 72%. It is possible that both conditions are related to thyroid function. They both respond after amalgam removal and I am just suggesting that thyroid may be one route of action to consider. Thyroid levels change, though.

Where do you find the problem? The famous T3 and T4? Maybe, but not necessarily. I look for changes in TSH, the thyroid stimulating hormone. TSH is present when the body requires more thyroid hormones. A person may have adequate levels of T3 and T4, but if the hormones are contaminated, for practical purposes the person is functionally thyroid deficient.

TSH is usually present in measurable amounts. A little is okay, but if the level is above one microgram (mcg), then I know that that person is functionally thyroid deficient. How much? This is related in a general way to the distance the level of TSH is above 1 mcg. It just tells me that the measurable thyroid hormones (T3 and T4) are in a good level, but that the hormones are contaminated and not functioning up to their proper capacity. The biochemically intelligent body is saying, regardless of the test level, I know that we are functionally deficient, therefore I am calling on the thyroid gland to make more hormone.

Emotions and Posterior Pituitary Hormones

Thyroid does not work alone in influencing emotions. The posterior pituitary hormone (oxytocin) joins forces with thyroid. It is difficult to tell which is more important in interpreting emotions, but based on clinical observations, the oxytocin may be slightly more influential. The Jarvis group used very small doses of posterior pituitary extract and could observe a change in a person's attitudes in one day. A patient of mine ran out of posterior pituitary extract on a weekend and called me at home for additional supplies. He had a family reunion coming up and wanted to be at his best. "It really makes that much difference?" I asked George, a salesman and former victim of depression. "I take that pill, and it changes the personality of the next 200 people I meet," he answered.

Blood pressure and hormones

Posterior pituitary hormone is really two hormones, oxytocin and vasopressin. The name vasopressin sounds like it might be related to vessel pressure. It is. High blood pressure is related to the function of the posterior pituitary gland. Since posterior pituitary activity is influenced by mercury, as well as thyroid hormone, and blood pressure is related to both, **do dental materials actually dictate where your blood pressure is?**

The pituitary gland is located just above the nasal sinus, just above the hard palate in the mouth. If you take the tip of your tongue and place it as far back on the roof of your mouth as you can, the posterior pituitary gland is about two inches above your tongue tip. It is not much of a trip for mercury vapor to leave a filling, travel into the sinus, and then travel about an inch through tissues to the pituitary gland.

Stortebecker showed that mercury from fillings could be detected in the thyroid glands of exposed dogs within less than a minute of amalgam placement in the dog's teeth. With the potential of the function of both the posterior pituitary and thyroid hormones being altered by mercury, we should be aware of this connection if we suffer from high blood pressure. Especially the type of high blood pressure that only minimally improves with drugs.

Suicide

If emotions are centered in the pituitary and thyroid glands, massive exposures to mercury vapor eight hours per day just might help explain why, as a profession, dentists rank highest in suicide. Autopsy studies in Sweden showed that the pituitary glands of dentists held 800 times more mercury than people who were not in dentistry. This is not surprising because dentists breathe in large amounts of mercury vapor while cutting out old amalgam fillings. When that drill, moving at 100,000 revolutions per minute, hits that amalgam filling, there is a massive amount of mercury vapor emitted.

Mercury is chemically called lipid soluble, which means soluble in fats. It therefore has the ability to enter cells through the fatty part of the cell membranes. It requires very little effort on the part of mercury to travel from the nasal cavity above the fillings up to the posterior pituitary gland.

Suicidal thoughts are not limited to dental personnel. I have been interested in suicidal tendencies for some years and have observed that over 90% of 2,000 of my patients had unexplained suicidal thoughts for no particular reason. Sure they were ill, but not that sick. That's a rather serious insinuation.

Specific gravity of the urine, or the weight of urine compared to that of water (1.000 by definition) is an indication of the function of our old emotional friend, the posterior pituitary gland. This is an indirect, inexpensive and highly accurate test for pituitary function developed by the Jarvis group.

When I found the specific gravity of the urine at levels below 1.008, I suspected that we had a strongly suicidal patient and I would openly discuss suicidal thoughts in a casual manner like it was a common occurrence. Easy, because it *was* common.

This subject had better be addressed before all others, however, for we could be sitting on potential disaster. If dental revision is not done properly, we could stimulate action that we did not need. These patients had to be under observation continually for twenty-four hours after the first amalgam removal—another connection between mercury and health potentials.

I have learned something I consider significant by talking to people who have come within seconds of suicide, then had something disturb the process. It may be surprising and gratifying to some people to learn that THE SUICIDAL ATTEMPTEES DID NOT REALIZE WHAT THEY WERE DOING. They kind of did, but the significance was lost. It was almost like: Should I tie my shoes, or shoot myself? Being of equal significance, which should I do first? Another gratifying point is that these unsolicited suicidal tendencies tend to disappear within a few days of dental revision—again, if it is done with respect to the protocol.

It really irritates me that suicide is close to the number-one cause of death in teenagers. I suggest that parents watch for personality changes that might occur within a few days of placement of braces. Braces increase the electrical and toxic load people are carrying if they have amalgam in their mouths. If their grades go down, and they change into a much different person from what they used to be, it might be well to know that they are potentially suicidal. Amalgam can create the suicidal problem by itself, but the addition of braces, nickel crowns, or even gold crowns evidently increases the exit rate of mercury, and the glands react. Or should I say, stop reacting?

It has been my observation that each teenager has a unique personality until reacting to mercury and other dental materials. After a certain point at which they undergo a change for the worse, they all have much more uniform behavior and personality. Mom and Dad, it's not your fault.

If this book does nothing more than reduce the teen suicide rate by generating awareness, it will have been worth the outrage toward this book that I anticipate from the uncaring dental associations and manufacturers.

Frequent or Nocturnal Urination

Although not a terminal disease, the problem of having to get up several times each night to urinate is disruptive to sleep, spouses, and one's general disposition. The center that controls this need is the posterior pituitary gland.

There is a certain amount of solid material that must be disposed of daily in the urine. If the concentration of these solids is high (yielding a specific gravity of 1.022 to 1.025) then the proper volume of urine will be excreted in a day. Should the concentration be half that, or yielding a specific gravity of 1.012 for instance, then it will take double the amount of urine to rid yourself of the same amount of solid. In other words, the solids remain the same. If the concentration of the urine is reduced, the total volume of urine is increased substantially. What controls the concentrating ability? The posterior pituitary gland.

Correction is not as simple as removing the amalgam. Yes, this will help, but maybe by reducing the nocturnal trips to the bathroom from four to two times a night. Dietary-wise, the more sugar and caffeine in the diet, the less the efficiency of the posterior pituitary gland. The Jarvis group found that after correcting the diet, if they gave a small amount of posterior pituitary extract, the nocturnal urination could be eliminated. Doses were prescribed according to the specific gravity readings. We found that by removing amalgam, the specific gravity could be improved. This was great, because it is difficult to find posterior pituitary extract in this country any more. The extract that I have found is not nearly as effective as what used to be available.

So, if one combines the dental revision with reduction of sugar and caffeine, there can be a notable improvement in both daytime frequency and nocturnal urination.

Menstrual Irregularities and Fertility

Many of the female fertility cycle events are related to posterior pituitary activity, so amalgam is another event that can disturb fertility as well as nonpregnant functions. Estrogen function can also be influenced by amalgam as seen working with the Jarvis group's techniques. Blood serum phosphorus was their guideline to endocrine balance. If the phosphorus was below 3.5 mg%, there was an endocrine disturbance, somewhat related to the degree of drop below 3.5. Low phosphorus did not tell which endocrine gland was out of balance, just that there was a disturbance.

Over the years, the Jarvis group found that the most effective hormones in balancing the phosphorus level were the sex hormones. They found that all males and all females produce both estrogen and testosterone. Obviously, the males produce more testosterone, and the females more estrogen, but there is a balance between the two in both sexes. Small doses of both hormones were used in both sexes (depending on the needs) to balance the serum phosphorus. When we discovered that amalgam removal alters endocrine function, it became apparent that without amalgam in the mouth, frequently *neither* hormone was required to balance the chemistry. This is not 100%, but more than 90% of the imbalances created by sex hormone disturbances corrected within a few weeks of amalgam removal.

We noted differences in fertility, less pain during periods, relief from endometriosis, and a trend toward optimization of the days of menstrual flow. It has been suggested that the uterus is a collection center for mercury. If that is true, it may explain what we see in a very high percentage of cases. We noted that most of the time the periods were six days or more prior to dental revision. Frequently the next period after dental revision was longer and heavier than usual. The resultant action we termed the "dental D&C." A D&C is the term for dilation of the cervix and curettage (or scraping out) of the uterus. If the dental removal procedures were finished around the time of the period, such that the body had three weeks until the next one, the following period was usually heavy. If dental revision was just in between the time of the periods, then this phenomenon did not show up until the next month. At any rate, the uterus responded to amalgam removal in particular by a massive housecleaning procedure, and after the month of heavy flow, the flow would usually approach four days.

Unaware of this, one thirty-two-year-old woman, who was confined to a nursing home with MS, had her amalgams removed. Her next period was heavy, so she was taken to the hospital and the doctors decided to perform a hysterectomy on her. This is not necessary. Just wait another month, and everything will probably be okay.

In extreme cases, we have noted that amenorrhea, or the complete absence of a menstrual flow, responds to amalgam removal. This is usually in women in their twenties or thirties. Even in women who have gone through a sort of premature menopause in their early forties, the periods may start up again for a couple of years. This has resulted in surprise pregnancies, so you should be informed.

Sterility in young males and females has been noted to change after total dental revision and complete balancing of the chemistries. Mother Nature does not like severe birth defects, and will stop the pregnancy process by multiple methods rather than deliberately allow a malformed child to be born. Temporary sterility is just one of them.

Just stepping over the boundary from nonfertility to fertility is not the whole story. We recommend that pregnancy be actively avoided, for at least six months after amalgam removal. Just stepping over the wire can still be in the arena of nonterminal birth defects. Now this brings up another interesting problem. You may remember from Chapter 2 that almost all lubricated condoms and birth control creams or gels have mercury as the primary spermicide. Since all of them contain mercury, it is unnecessary for the word mercury to appear on the label, for everyone knows mercury is in there. Right? If you are planning a pregnancy, you should really be informed of this exposure and use a non-mercury method.

Estrogen and Testosterone

As has been shown by monitoring the actual serum levels of estrogen and testosterone in both males and females, there can be dramatic changes in both levels after amalgam removal. The fallout from changing these hormones can create alterations in everything from personalities to blood pressure to fertility and probably dozens of other symptoms that encourage people to seek help from their doctors. PMS is one of the most common symptoms to see change after amalgam removal.

Diabetes

Diabetes has multiple contributing factors. Genetics is but one. Dr. Ralph Steinman once told me that diabetes was so hereditary that it occurred in families whether the children were adopted or natural. "Whattt???" I had asked.

"It all depends on what the family eats for breakfast," he answered. Steinman had found that excessive carbohydrate intake for breakfast was significantly related to the onset of diabetes.

Insulin, the molecule of question in diabetes, has three sulfur binding sites. Should mercury attach to one of these . . . same old story: interference with normal biological function.

Blood sugar, or glucose as it is called chemically, is one of the chemistries that we monitor during dental revision. In the complete program, we alter people's diets as well as their fillings, so one cannot relate mercury to the whole change. Glucose did change notably, however. In diabetics the daily requirements for insulin usually dropped to less than half what they had been before dental revision. Most of the diabetics we treated monitored their blood sugar levels several times a day. We recommend this for diabetics because insulin requirements can change after dental revision and insulin overdoses can occur. Be informed. If you are taking insulin, watch your sugar levels.

References for this Chapter

Jarvis Group. Collected correspondance between D. C. Jarvis and numerous letter-writers. Information collected and evaluated between 1920 and 1950 by Jarvis, who disseminated findings to group.

Nylander, M., L. Friberg, D. Eggleston, L. Bjorkman. 1989. Mercury accumulation in tissues from dental staff and controls in relation to exposure. *Swedish Dental Journal* 13:235-243.

Stortebecker, Patrick. 1982. *Dental Caries as a Cause of Nervous Disorders.* Sweden: Stortebecker Foundation for Research.

Steinman, R. R., et al. December 1963. A demonstration of human food combinations upon dental caries. *Journal of the Southern California State Dental Association*, vol. 31, no. 12.

PART II

Disease Responses Seen after Dental Revision

8

Diseases that Respond to Dental Revision
or
Observations of the Incurable

There are a number of diseases that respond to dental revision. Most of them required fairly complex forms of treatment to bring about a response, but if the total protocol was used, we did see an amazing number of reversals. Back in the mid 1970s, we felt elated if we saw a response in some of these diseases 10% of the time. With the advent of the multidisciplined approach, that figure gradually climbed to over 80% response.

Many diseases have a unique trigger that initiates the healing process. The entire protocol may have an effect, but healing does not really get into action until the unique trigger is released. Where a trigger exists, or where I (HH) have stumbled onto it, it will be described.

I am gratified to hear almost every week from other areas of the country where dental and medical groups are joining together to fight the establishment and develop better methods of treating patients. It is illegal for physicians and dentists to practice together for mutual patient benefit, because one board cannot censure all folks who work there. Many of these groups are trying to duplicate the basic concepts of multidisciplined treatment we had in Colorado Springs before the wise judges and board of dental examiners proclaimed that mercury was perfectly safe and Huggins was out of line to say it is not. So far, the closest practice is that of Dr. Javier Morales, now in Puerto Vallarta, Mexico. I help train the physicians, dentists, and other personnel in our concepts, and do I love the mystic jungle environment—especially in the winter. Summer, well that's another story for a Colorado boy.

In the meantime, here is what can be, and has been, accomplished. You should be informed. If you can avoid having mercury, nickel, and root canals placed, you may not require the services of a system like what Huggins Diagnostic provided.

Fibromyalgia

Fibromyalgia is basically pain. Where? All over more than any place else. I don't think I had even heard the word fifteen years ago, and now we get requests for referrals several times each week. It is becoming more popular all the time.

This is another one of those complex issues. The dietary changes, supplementation, amalgam removal, etc., must be done as a matter of course to set up the body for recovery. The usual dental revision techniques are not the whole story, however. In many diseases of dental origin as I mentioned, there is a unique trigger that must be addressed. In the case of fibromyalgia, it is often condensing osteitis.

If the body is fighting a losing battle with an infected tooth, it will try to wall off the offending tooth rather than let the infection run rampant through the body. This wall-ing off of the tooth is accomplished by forming a dense calcium layer around the tooth. This frequently happens with a root canal tooth. The extra thickening of calcium gives an X-ray the appearance of a well-healed tooth in which healthy cementum is forming. It is actually not healing at all. The area immediately surrounding the tooth is building an armor plate to prevent the sick tooth from infecting the whole body.

Condensing osteitis is so dense that it easily overshadows abscesses and cysts on the tooth and gives the appearance of an "X-ray negative tooth." After a tooth with condensing osteitis is extracted by conventional methods, future X-rays will show the outline of the tooth. I used to see these and think, "there is the outline of the tooth." Nothing else would cross my mind. Little did I realize that what I was seeing was a dense calcium cone that was filled, not with healed bone, but with infected materials, necrotic bone and anaerobic bacteria with their waste products.

This condensing osteitis must be removed with a dental surgical burr along with about a millimeter of what would appear to be sound bone surrounding it. The same procedure is used that is employed in removing the ligament around a root canal tooth after the tooth is extracted. The entire technique involves using a round burr, lots of sterile water and vacuum, flush with a nonvasoconstricting anesthetic, and protamine zinc insulin for accelerated healing.

The most outstanding example of rapid response I ever saw was that of a woman whose husband was a medical doctor. He had sent her to everyone he could think of, and still she had been in constant pain for three years. All three molars on the lower right side had been removed, and the condensing osteitis outlines were clearly visible on X-ray. As the dentist was cutting out the second molar osteitis lining, she sighed and announced that the pain had just stopped for the first time in three years. She never again experienced the discomfort of fibromyalgia.

But remember, it is not just removing the osteitis, not just the diet, not just anything. The whole package must be utilized, and sometimes then, it is not enough.

Epilepsy

There are evidently several types of seizure activity. A neurologist was in our office one time observing videos of patients. One patient was having violent seizures, and the doctor announced that she did not have epilepsy. "What do you call this if it is not epilepsy?" I asked. "I don't know," he answered, "but she is conscious for the first part of the seizure activity. In epilepsy, the patient is unconscious."

About half of our patients were conscious during most of their seizure activity in the dental chair. The scenario was quite predictable. Here is how it reads: Dental personnel were aware of the potential, so were alert to upcoming events. The unique trigger in seizure activity is that the fillings have to be removed in *absolute* sequence, and not by quadrant. This means remove the highest single negative filling first, then the second highest filling, even if it is in a different quadrant. Sometimes, when the final milligram of the first filling is removed, the patient will probably have a twenty-second—more or less—seizure, and that may be their last. The seizures are seldom violent unless the patient is normally having ten to twenty seizures a day. Yes, we have seen twenty seizures per day in people who could not tolerate taking the normal medications.

The worst-case scenario in improvement occurs in people with multiple seizures daily, even on heavy medication. They may be reduced to one or two seizures per day, but not stop completely. They have been elated to have this much reduction, so it was never a problem, but seizures do not always go away completely. The important thing is that they might not ever have had seizures if they had never been exposed to dental toxins.

One of our patients, a 5'10" female with the most admirable attitude I have ever seen, was having more than ten grand mal seizures a day. Considering her size and strength, the seizures were highly destructive to any human or furniture within reach. She was a human flailing machine at these times. Removing her first filling elicited a twenty-second seizure (which is typical) and six of us were in the dental operatory, prepared to do whatever the situation dictated. She was more expressive in seizure activity than most people, but with the removal of the first filling, the seizure was quite mild by comparison with her normal seizure behavior.

In her case, it was elected to use acupressure for fifteen minutes just prior to dental removal of that first, highest negatively charged amalgam. That seemed to help, so it became routine with severe seizure patients to utilize acupressure therapy just prior to the first dental appointment, but after the anesthetic was administered.

After she returned home seizure-free, her physician decided that this was just a temporary cessation of activity, and that she needed a strong antibiotic to keep her in this spontaneous remission. She took the antibiotic and within a few hours returned to multiple seizures every day for over a week. Makes you wonder about just what antibiotics do besides kill bacteria.

Can acupressure be considered another unique trigger in the cessation of seizure activity? I don't know, but I do recommend that it be utilized if possible. Another questionable trigger is that the patients were seen in the Bubble operatory.

This is a giant bubble-shaped room that is surrounded by a Faraday cage. The cage reduces the electrical bombardment that is usually present due to radio and TV waves, cellular phone communications, satellite movie projections, and the dozens of other forms of radiant energy present.

Fillings are pushing very high electrical charges into the brain relative to what the brain normally operates on, and it is felt that removal of the high charges could alter compensatory brain function. I liken it to walking into a seventy-mile-an-hour windstorm. If you lean forward hard enough, you can do it. But what if the wind suddenly stops? You will fall on your face. Possibly when the electrical charge stops as the last milligram of amalgam is removed, you not only are faced with stopping the compensation, but are susceptible to other electrical currents. A lot of suppositions, but neurological patients, and epilepsy patients in particular, recover notably better in the cage than in the operatory we used before we had the Bubble operatory.

We have had reports that people with epilepsy have had follow-up electroencephalograms (EEGs) performed after going home. If improvement stays with them, the interferences in the EEG seem to disappear. If the brain operates on 6 to 9 nanoamperes of current, and fillings are bombarding the brain with up to 100 or more microamperes, it should be no surprise that brain function could improve when the excessive electrical current is removed. You have a right to be informed.

Arthritis

Arthritis is in the category of autoimmune diseases, or diseases in which one's own immune system begins to destroy one's own tissues. From a dental standpoint, arthritis could be stimulated by any of the immunoreactive dental materials, which include not only amalgam, but nickel crowns and root canals as well.

Dental materials may initiate the activity, but there are other things that continue the activity and even make it worse, even after the fillings have been replaced. One of the unique triggers in arthritis is orange juice. Oranges themselves will do the same thing. Usually arthritics drink orange juice at least five times a week. Each shot of juice will give you a good attack for four days, so there is no stopping the pain of arthritis (without drugs) as long as the juice habit is continued.

Caffeine is another trigger. Amalgam removal will start the trend toward improvement for a few days due to the immune stimulation that occurs when fillings are removed. A week or two later the same old symptoms will recur. There is a lot more to the protocol, but do the protocol and continue coffee (or caffeine in any form) or orange juice, and I offer a written guarantee that you will never improve.

What happens when orange juice and caffeine enter the system? There is a relationship between calcium and phosphorus normally found in the bloodstream. According to Dr. Page and the Jarvis group, calcium and phosphorus form a compound that floats around in the bloodstream looking for bone to build. When something elevates the calcium or lowers the phosphorus, calcium is liberated from this compound. Calcium will not remain liberated and uncombined for very long, so it will usually combine with a substance like sulfates or oxides that will precipitate. If this calcium precipitates in the joints, it contributes to arthritis. The area of precipitation is usually under genetic direction, for there are multiple tissues into which calcium can precipitate.

The body also has a continual degeneration-regeneration cycle. Red blood cells are a good example. A red blood cell lives for 120 days, then must be recycled, or degenerated. A new one is regenerated in its place. If the two cycles were absolutely equal, we would live forever, so obviously we degenerate some every day. Orange juice and caffeine accelerate the degeneration cycle and slow the regeneration cycle. Any time we take these substances into our bodies, we are accelerating our breakdown process. Arthritis is an example of a degenerative disease and anything that accelerates the degenerative cycle will make arthritis get worse.

What about those nodules on the knuckles of people with longstanding arthritis? They may reduce in size a tad over the years after amalgam removal, but that has little to do with function. Even large-knuckled folks can notice tremendous improvements in finger function within weeks, with absolutely no change in knuckle size. It's okay for you to be informed. Arthritis may not be an ibuprofen deficiency.

Do the *Eyes* Have It? Well, They Get It.

It is well documented in the scientific literature that visual disturbances are one of the early signs of mercury intoxication. There is evidence that visual disturbances can be created in utero.

Dr. Doty Murphy pointed out that he could see black areas in the retinas of the eyes of people with amalgams that were not there in people who were amalgam-free. He had also observed that when these black areas were present, the person was nearsighted. He had noticed this in children in particular. After baby teeth with amalgam fell out, there was a gradual disappearance of the black areas.

This started a long series of sessions with a local ophthalmologist who owned a special "fundus photography" type of camera. We soon found, usually but not always, a crescent-shaped black area around the optic disc on the retina. According to the textbooks, these areas occurred in nearsighted people because the eye had elongated, and the underlying epithelium was showing through. These books did not address the fact that the black areas go away after amalgam removal.

When did you start wearing glasses? I did when I was sixteen. When did you have your first amalgam placed? I did when I was sixteen. I have asked this question of hundreds of audiences and find that roughly 40% of the people who can remember these two events had both occur within the same year.

I even startled my eye doctor by having over half of my astigmatism disappear when I was fifty years old. That was a year after I stopped removing amalgam. I found that I could hire dentists to do that. We protected them with all kinds of devices in the Bubble operatory, but that is still not like being totally away from mercury vapor. I was having a particularly hard time with turning fifty, so I remember the event well. He told me he was surprised to see that happen—"especially in a man of your age." Oh, did that hurt.

I had mentioned the eye changes and showed slides of the changes to a medical audience in Paris in the late '80s. In the late '90s, I gave another lecture to another medical audience in Paris. This time a lady eye doctor interrupted me and made some excited remarks from the audience. The moderator told her to come up on the stage and bring her slides. It seems that after hearing me some years before, she had begun recommending amalgam removal in people with severe eye problems. She spent twenty minutes showing slides and giving vivid verbal descriptions (in

French) about the changes that she had observed in her patients. The audience was thoroughly impressed. I could see the fundus photography changes in the retinas, but unfortunately could not understand a word she said.

You have a right to think about your eyes the next time your dentist insists on placing amalgam.

For Whom the Bell's Palsy Tolls

I have seen what I thought was a relationship between Bell's Palsy and mercury, but nothing as vivid as the onset related to placement of a nickel crown. The dentist is apt to tell you it is a porcelain crown and forget to announce that the porcelain was fired onto a nickel thimble that was cast to fit your tooth. The metal composition is always downplayed unless it is really gold. Today the majority of the ceramic or porcelain crowns are fired onto nickel; another way of evading the subject is to call it "nonprecious" metal crown material.

Just removing the crown is not the secret, as I am sure you know now. The unique trigger in remission of Bell's Palsy is the Feldenkrais method. Feldenkrais is a body discipline that helps reintroduce the nervous system to the muscular system. Exercises that stimulate the redevelopment of these nerve-muscle pathways can be very effective after nickel crown removal—if all the dietary and mineral imbalances are being addressed simultaneously. You have the right to know that cancer is not the only disturbance that nickel produces.

Breast Cancer

It would be hard to see the connection between a police department and breast cancer, but that's where it started.

I was asked by a police department that shall remain nameless, with the exception of "PD," to offer information on the toxicity of nickel in crowns. It seems that a certain dentist had a lifestyle that was way beyond his means, and PD was looking for an explanation. The answer was found in that said dentist was placing and billing for thousands of "gold" crowns. According to the analysis of the crowns, there was no gold, but lots of other strange metals. Nickel was the primary one. Further investigation found that these samples of nonprecious metal varied slightly in composition. The variation was discovered to depend on whether they originally came from Volkswagen, Pontiac, or Oldsmobile bumpers in the junkyard. What an insult. I thought there was more quality control than that to nonprecious dental metals. There probably is with some companies; but, is it necessary to have quality control for toxins?

Somehow the investigation centered on a cul-de-sac that housed twenty families in their twenties and thirties We were looking for nickel crowns. We found that the first woman interviewed had just had surgery for intraductal carcinoma of the breast. A second woman, who lived next door, had just been operated on and intraductal carcinoma was also found on microscopic pathology examination. A few houses yielded nothing of significance, then another young woman with—yes, the same tumor. Within a half day, the investigation turned up six women under the age of forty with identical breast tumors. That's highly unusual to find such a concentration of the identical tumor in women so young. Breast cancer is a disease of the forties and fifties, and up. Not twenties. Interesting that they all went to the same dentist, all had the same type of nickel-ceramic crown with metal from the same junkyard laboratory. Suspicious?

Remember reading the nickel section? What does nickel do consistently? It generates cancer. Is there a relationship? Since that little investigation (fraud charges against the dentist were dropped), I have asked lots of women who were diagnosed with breast cancer if they had nickel-ceramic crowns. Not a scientific study, but if I were female and had a desire to maintain all my body parts, I don't believe I would subject myself to the challenge of nickel-ceramic crowns.

A professor in a large university on the East Coast told me that if I wanted to study fluoride and tooth decay, he could get me a million-dollar grant with no problem. But, if the research had anything to do with mercury or nickel—especially dealing with cancer—there was no way he could furnish even one dime.

According to the work of Dr. Joseph Issels of Germany, when he treated breast cancer, he had a dentist remove all the patient's root canals before he started. He saw a direct relationship between the two. If you really want to be safe, I suppose you should consider both root canals and nickel if you have a family history of breast cancer. Think twice if you are given dental advice regarding the need for root canals and nickel-porcelain crowns. Isn't this worth a major scientific "study"? Could be that one might be done by the year 3000. You have a right to know about my observations now, and the supporting evidence, then you may make up your own mind.

But—if you have had a nickel chrome crown as a child, braces later on, or as an adult had a nickel removable partial denture, a root canal and breast cancer, lumps, or fibrocystic disease of the breast—would you please write to me and describe your situation? Maybe with a few thousand letters, a private foundation will get interested. Don't expect help from the establishment. Too many lawsuits could result from this information if it turned out to be the primary cause of breast cancer.

The only unique trigger I found here was the initiating factor of nickel-porcelain crowns. Additionally root canals may be a compounding trigger factor. Too many people demonstrate these correlations. Just be informed, and inform me of your consequences.

Parkinson's Disease

My mother died of Parkinson's, so I have always had a personal vendetta against the disease. When she came down with it, I looked for disturbances in her chemistries. I found them. Better than that, I knew how to correct every one of the imbalances. The only problem was that it didn't work.

That was eight years before I spotted the trigger for healing. Cavitations. Cavitations are those areas of incomplete healing where a tooth has been removed. Cavitations most often occur (around 90% of the time) in the wisdom tooth areas, but theoretically they can occur in any extraction site. Cavitations are described in detail in chapter 12.

In Parkinson's disease, if everything is followed in the protocol—with the exception of cleaning out the cavitations, nothing happens. Maybe a little something. Chemistries do improve, but nothing of real physical significance occurs. Follow the protocol *and* clean the cavitations, and many steps toward recovery can occur. The disease doesn't go away entirely except in a few cases, but the basic symptoms of tremors can be improved far greater than 50%. The improvements have been gratifying. I only wish I had been informed twenty years ago.

E.I.

Now called "chemically sensitive," the formerly "environmentally ill" (or before that "Universal Reactor") patient lives a miserable life. So does everyone in the same family or household. It is a frustrating disease because you don't even get to wear a band-aid. It doesn't show for the most part and the patient's reactions to common substances in the environment are so severe that most people believe that their problem is "all in their head."

We built our office for the E.I. patient. I figured that if an E.I. could handle it, anyone could. We spend thousands of extra dollars to get drywall without mercury, nonoutgassing carpet cement, paint without mercury (don't believe what they tell you), and dozens of other "little" things that chemically sensitive people react to. After the second E.I. patient had seizures in the reception room, I decided that a perfectly clean entire office could not be achieved practically.

These folks loved the Bubble operatory, for the air and environment in there were really super, first-class. But that one room cost $100,000 to build. I was severely criticized by the Colorado attorney general for charging people to be in such a needlessly clean room. She dropped the subject when it was discovered that I donated the room to patients. They didn't have to pay anything extra to be treated in a clean environment. It was my experiment and my gift. It worked. It was worth it.

What goes on in the body of a chemically sensitive person? Bedlam. Their immune system overreacts to about everything except cotton and wood. The whole idea of working with chemically sensitive people was cemented in my mind back in 1983. We were treating a patient who was sensitive to just about everything. She and her husband would sit in their car until we were ready to perform something, then rush in, be treated, and rush out. There were no filling materials that her body could handle, so we were taking out fillings and leaving the teeth bare. Sounds bizarre, but it gave her a life back. After one year, she could tolerate a certain filling material, so her teeth were restored to normal.

The first day of her amalgam removal was particularly hectic. Not only did I have many life-threatening incidents with her, but it seemed like everyone in the country who dialed 911 got my office. I had started early in the morning, missed lunch, and at 9:30 P.M. was finally able to leave the office. I was the most put-upon person in the world. There is nothing like missing two meals to make you feel that way. Plus, it had snowed four inches and I was going to have to clean snow off the car and windshield before rushing to reach a restaurant before it closed.

Then I got my commitment. Their car was parked next to mine. As I cleaned the snow off my car, I could not help but notice two body forms bundled up on clothless springs that used to be car seats. They could not go to a motel due to the massive number of things she reacted to. She mentioned that their car had to be stripped to the bare bones, but I was not prepared for what I saw. Even the ceiling and doors had all the upholstery removed.

And I was put upon? Tears rolled down my cheeks as I scraped the snow from the windows and slid onto my luxurious leather seats. What kind of life do dentists inflict on some patients without even knowing it? Her problems had started just after having about twelve new high-copper fillings placed in one week. I suppose I ate dinner that night. I don't remember. But I have never felt "put upon" since that experience.

I compare the chemically sensitive patient's immune system to an experience I call the cat story. I had a cat. I liked the cat, and the cat liked me. One day the cat got into an argument with the dog next door. I rushed out and picked up the cat. Cat interpreted me as dog, and proceeded to make stripes out of my flesh. She was so upset with that dog that everything looked like a dog. The E.I. patient's immune system reacts to everything that has a protein antigen. Their system is not really tuned in to everything on the planet as nonself, but it reacts like it feels that way.

It takes very careful treatment and lots of time to improve the E.I. patient. What I didn't like was that many of them did not want to get better. Who wouldn't like to crawl out of that abyss? The control freak. There are some people who have never been in a position of authority, and find comfort in being able to say, "Oh, you have on aftershave—please go wash it off or I will have a violent reaction." (And it will be your fault, guilt trip, guilt trip.) "Wash your clothes with this soap, or I cannot be around you." None of our personnel were allowed to wear anything scented and we paid particular attention to cleaning supplies, etc., etc., etc., yet the E.I. patient would still complain bitterly. When I found that these same folks would order pizza with all sorts of offensive things on it, and desserts that would set their chemistries into orbit just to make up for their miserable lifestyle, I rethought the situation. If two were in the office at one time, they competed to see which one was worse off. After a year of this, we limited the visits of E.I. patients to one per month.

Is that unkind? They were so disruptive to the patients who wanted to get well that we developed an intensive screening program, and I wrote a song. Sung to the tune of Old McDonald's Farm, it went "E.I., E.I. NO!" With our new screening program in place, we found to our delight that there were E.I. patients who were willing to take responsibility for the long arduous trip toward improvement. Not getting completely well, just improvement.

The unique trigger for the E.I. patient was time, patience, and an enormous amount of discipline. It took several months to see positive improvements, and the slightest infraction would set them back a month or more. After a year, things would look pretty good. They could go to the grocery store—downtown for half an hour at a time—as long as they stayed far away from the perfume counters. After three years, they could live a reasonably pleasant life, but still had to be cautious to avoid known chemical exposures. E.I. patients probably work harder for less improvement than any other dentally oriented patients I have seen. It's not for everybody. You have to be really tough and disciplined to improve. The really sad part to me, though, is that it didn't have to happen. Almost all the patients we saw could directly connect a dental event to the onset of their problems. If only they had known. That's why you have a right to know.

Allergies

Allergies are the stepchild of the chemically sensitive person. There are many dietary initiators for allergies because of the way in which the immune system individually handles each challenge. When additional immune insult is added with mercury, nickel, copper, and other metals in dental materials, allergies can get worse. It is not easy to separate the chicken from the egg in allergy origination, but it can be observed that each immune issue enhances the other, such that the combination produces allergy.

Getting rid of the metal immune reactors can improve allergies, but there is no trigger I have noted here except that all avenues must be covered to gain moderate success.

Red and White Blood Cells

Red army

Red and white blood cells are really first cousins, although they don't look much alike on close examination. White blood cells have a nucleus. In fact, they have several different types of nuclei ranging from occupying almost all of the internal space of the cell to only about half of it. Red blood cells, on the other hand, have no nucleus at all. Whites have all kinds of enzymes within them that are weapons of mass destruction for bacteria and other invading forces that might get into our bodies. Red cells contain hemoglobin for the transport of oxygen, and that's about all they do most of the time.

But they both come from the same parents, called stem cells. They are both susceptible to challenges from mercury. Here they differ, primarily because of their functional duties.

When red blood cells become contaminated with mercury, they have less ability to transport oxygen. To compensate for this, they increase in numbers to have more potential to carry oxygen. If they really start producing lots and lots of "extra" cells, the red count looks like the disease called hemoconcentration. This refers to an excessive amount of cells per volume, which leads to molasses-type blood. It is like too many cars on the freeway. The original idea was to provide more transportation, but a cellular logjam occurs in which the actual overall movement slows down. The patient's face may be dark purple—especially in the cheeks, and the men are said to have a "ruddy" complexion.

The unique trigger in correcting this disorder is to add potassium. Not just any potassium (certainly not "lite" salt, or sea salt), but one that is in a highly absorbable form. Some people have had to have bloodletting done every few months to keep the red cell count down, and the blood is considered "contaminated" and not worthy of transfusion. No one has ever given a reason except for fear of the unknown. What made it go up in the first place? Is it "catching"? I doubt it is catching, for the high cell count seems to be a compensation for mercury contamination. You have a right to know that hemoconcentration appears to be a defense mechanism for contamination from your fillings, and that you are really okay.

White army

White blood cells have a different role to play in reacting to mercury exposure. This explanation may be a little deep for most people, but for doctors who may be interested in how dentistry influences their patient's immune systems, it might be worth a page to explain what is happening.

White blood cells come in what is called "populations." There are roughly six types of cells in most people, but there can be more in the leukemic. The rest are my observations. Unchallenged people with no amalgam, or those who are not otherwise exposed to immunoreactive materials, will have only lymphocytes and polymorphonuclear leukocytes (PMNs). Their total white cell count will be between 5,000 and 6,000 cells per cubic millimeter. If they are really pure, the count will be between 5,000 and 5,500.

When amalgam (or probably nickel and root canals because of the similarity of immune reactivity) is (are) placed, the PMNs increase, the lymphocytes decrease, and the total white cell count will increase from 1,000 to 3,000. Unless, of course, one is super healthy. In these cases, the whites may go up even higher until the condition is called leukemia. (Again, remember, this is Huggins' opinion, based on several decades of observation.)

PMNs are the first to war with mercury exposure, and they engulf as much as they can. Not being able to destroy mercury, the cell malfunctions due to mercury messing up its internal chemistry, and the cell erupts and dies. Its contents chemically signal the other immune cells that we are losing the war, and to send heavy artillery. The body supplies monocytes in response to that request. These fighters are far more effective than the foot soldier PMNs. They are more like a foot soldier with a bazooka.

Monocytes come onto the scene and fight for a while until it is obvious that they cannot destroy mercury, either. As they approach about 6% or 7% of the fighting force, they signal for their backup cells, the Sherman tanks of the immune fighting force called the eosinophils. Eos join the fracas until at 3% or 4% of the total warriors, it is evident that they cannot destroy mercury either, so they signal for their backup, the basophils. Basos represent the atomic warheads of the battle.

When Basos can't contain the event, either, the extra fighters retire rather than deplete all their backup reserves, for they require lots of fuel to maintain their fighting status, and the war system reverses. Basos disappear, then eos disappear except for maybe 1%, monos reduce their forces to 2% or 3%, and the total drops from the initial 3,000 to 5,000 increase to nearly normal, then over a period of months, maybe years, will finally slip below the 5,000 mark to 4,000 or even 3,000.

Sometime during this recession of troops, the fatigued immune system begins to send in untrained troops—often referred to as the children—to do a man's job of fighting. These guys are known as "bands" or "stabs." They look like fighters, but are so immature they do not have guns or any other weapons with which to fight. To me, 1% or 2% indicates that a noteworthy challenge is present. Let's not wait to find out why we died, let's identify the challenge and eliminate it.

It is Huggins' opinion that the reason the "normal" or average range seen in hospitals has changed so much over the past ten or fifteen years is to accommodate the reactions created by the high-copper amalgams. It used to be that practically no hospital had normals listed below 5,000 cells per cubic millimeter. Now some are approaching 3,000 or less as normal. The high end has been pushed up to 11,000 and 11,500 in some cases. Even bands have moved from the old 0% to 2% up to 2% to 11%. Today if you have no bands, you are considered abnormal.

From this scenario, you can see that the two systems, the healthy unchallenged system and the fatigued system, can strongly resemble each other at one time during the battle. There is one difference, however. At the rest (unchallenged) condition around 5,000, the lymphocytes will comprise about 2,400 of the total 5,000. During fatigue, the lymphocytes will only be about 1,400 to 1,600 of the 5,000. Aside from that, they do look much alike. Here is where the doctor must be astute and take an in-depth look at the patient. Numbers do not tell everything. If the patient looks and acts healthy, that may be true. If the patient looks like death warmed over, that may be true. Most of the patients we saw were in the latter category, but because their chemistries were within the new (wider) normal ranges, they were told by their doctors that their problems were "all in their head."

Removal of the offending dental materials starts a whole new alteration of percentages of cell changes, but that is not within the scope of informing you of the problems. Sequential removal is important also, or the healing trends will not be seen. But that is treatment, not informing you of the potential problems. The point here is that you deserve to be informed that the dental materials in your mouth can have a great influence on your immune system and your ability to fight off any challenges.

Systemic Lupus Erythematosus (SLE)

Lupus is classified as a terminal autoimmune disease, even though it may take many years to actually cause death. Lupus is a disease in which the nucleus of the cell is attacked. In theory, I suppose it could attack any cell, but lupus has a definite affinity for kidney cells. After becoming comfortable in its kidney home, the target selection may extend to the skin, joints, and heart.

Lupus is diagnosed by identifying antibodies called antinuclear antibodies (ANA) in the bloodstream. The term used in diagnosis is titer, or to be specific, the ANA titer. An example of very low reactivity would be an ANA titer of 1:60, spoken as "a titer of one to sixty." The higher the second number, the more severe the disease.

In theory, disease is gone if the titer drops to zero. That is not supposed to happen, but we have seen it drop in almost every case, and achieve zero more than half the time. Challenging. The most severe case we treated had a titer of 1:6400, which is astronomical. Reviewing her five-year history, she dropped to zero in less than six months (faster than usual), then went through a pregnancy with no titer reappearing, and is still zero six years after delivery. Not bad.

Symptoms that are noticeable include extra sensitivity to light, a characteristic skin rash over the nose and cheeks, kidney disorders, occasional nerve disorders including seizures and psychoses, blood disorders leaning toward anemia, and low white blood cell and platelet counts.

Treatment usually consists of taking the drug prednisone. This is the proverbial rock-and-hard-place situation, for prednisone is especially destructive to the lupus patient, but is the only drug found to "control" the disease.

Hultman and Enestrom in 1988 published research demonstrating that 1.6 milligrams (thousandths of a gram) of mercury injected into mice twice a week for four weeks produced ANA antibodies in 99% of the mice tested. Special testing called immunofluorescence revealed that no other autoantibodies were formed except the mercury-induced ANA antibodies.

Frequency of occurrence of lupus in the U.S. is approximately one per 2,000 people.

I became interested in lupus for two reasons. It had a measurable gauge, the ANA titer, and it seemed to respond readily to our protocol of treatment. After monitoring patients for a few years, I began to wonder if there were a relationship between the metals reactivity we studied in compatibility testing and the presence of titers. Compatibility testing is an immune test of how reactive a patient's serum is to each of the ninety-plus ingredients in dental materials. About twenty of these compatibility tests are for metals. I noted that the lupus patients had quite high reactivities to mercury, copper, and zinc. What segment of our population is most often exposed to mercury? Dental personnel gets my vote. What is the frequency of occurrence in the general population? One in 2,000.

I ran ANA titers on a series of twenty-five dentists to see if I could find one with a titer. Statistically it was foolish to even think of finding one in twenty-five who would have an ANA titer, with probability telling me one in 2,000 was the anticipated average. I did have an advantage, though. I tested only dentists who were highly reactive to mercury, copper, and zinc. That was the majority of them.

Amalgam consists of all of these metals, and a dentist who cuts out an amalgam exposes all his personnel and himself to the vapors of all these metals, so high reactivity was not a surprise. The titers were low, 1:60 up to 1:160, in which few if any problems would draw attention to themselves as symptoms. Not only did I find one, I found thirteen out of the twenty-five to have ANA titers. That 50%, as compared with an anticipated 0.05%, looked somewhat implicating toward sensitivities to the combination of mercury, copper, and zinc. This sort of a pattern appears in Alzheimer's too, as you will see if you read that section. If I were a "wet-finger" dentist, as the saying goes, I believe I would think twice if I had this information.

Haley Links Amalgam to Alzheimer's

Hollywood producer John Woods told me one day that I should meet Dr. Boyd Haley of the University of Kentucky. The same day he told Haley that he should meet Dr. Hal Huggins of Colorado Springs. We finally made telephone connection, and I began to tell Dr. Haley about the changes we were seeing in Alzheimer's patients after dental revision. Now, it is helpful to understand that Dr. Haley is one of the most highly published, highly respected, nitpicky orthodox scientists that ever walked the planet. He was also investigating Alzheimer's from a highly scientific protocol—and probably somewhat protective of his turf. Here's this small-town dentist telling him about Alzheimer's. Only due to his gentlemanly manner and respect for our mutual friend did he even take the time to listen to me.

Mercury related to Alzheimer's, yes, Haley had already done preliminary investigations there, and yes, there could be a possible connection. But hadn't the ADA researched the security of mercury in amalgam—by the way, how do you know there is mercury in amalgam? But root canals? No way. What could possibly be a problem there? That's just a tooth.

Just to be nice, or, as Haley later told me, to find a scientific way to shut up this guy Huggins, Haley tested the materials being generated in root canal teeth.

Two critical proteins are involved in brain function. These are tubulin and creatine kinase. Haley's biochemical laboratory at the university had already shown that the major difference in an Alzheimer's brain and a non-Alzheimer's brain was that the activity of tubulin and creatine kinase were greatly reduced in Alzheimer's brains.

Imagine his shock when a small amount of solution prepared by soaking two extracted root canal teeth in water totally obliterated both tubulin and creatine kinase. Haley called me and asked what was in a root canal that could be that toxic. I had no idea; in fact, that's why I had asked for his help.

He asked for more teeth to test. We supplied bunches of them, as did other interested dentists. In addition to the extracted teeth, we had all of the blood information, medical and dental history, etc., that were used in our dental revision protocol. Haley found that microliter amounts of water in which teeth had been soaked caused death of these proteins in brains and in separate purified individual tests. He then monitored time and found that in the presence of these root canal toxins, it took only a few minutes to inactivate tubulin and creatine kinase significantly. He was beside himself. "This stuff is extremely toxic. It definitely doesn't belong in humans."

Haley was amazed at the thoroughness of the testing Dr. Weston Price had done in the 1920s, when he was head of research for the American Dental Association. Few researchers today are as meticulous as Price and his staff of Ph.D.s.

Haley had developed a radioactive method of labeling proteins that far exceeded the sensitivity of any other method used today. His work in Alzheimer's indicated that the ability of tubulin and creatine kinase to perform their normal tasks in these patients are far below where they should be for proper brain function. Tubulin acts like a scaffold within our cells that gives each cell its form. Without tubulin, the cell collapses and becomes nonfunctional.

One of the basic purposes of digesting food is to furnish blood sugar for the brain. The brain is the number one most important organ in the body, and as such has many protective devices surrounding it. The skull and the blood-brain barrier are two of the most obvious. Creatine kinase is important for transferring cellular energy from one site to another. This unidentified root canal chemical inactivated creatine kinase.

Data was already available that mercury provided the same type of inactivation. I was interested to learn what Haley had discovered about mercury, because we had seen slow, but constant, improvements in Alzheimer's patients after dental revision and use of our protocol.

Haley had found that mercury at 1 to 5 micromolar concentrations (that's super-double-plus low) would totally abolish the activity of tubulin—and here is the important part—without any noticeable effect on other brain proteins. That had already been published. Why are we sitting on such valuable information while placing tons (literally) of mercury in people's mouths? Especially why are we placing the high-copper amalgams that release 50 times more mercury than the older versions of amalgam?

Then Haley wondered if any other metals would do the same thing that mercury did in deactivating his two favorite proteins. He tested about twenty metals and found that lead, cadmium, and zinc had some effect, but nothing aside from these even approached inactivating these proteins the way mercury did.

About this time, Haley found an article on the cytotoxic activity in solutions in which dental amalgams had been soaked. It stated that cytotoxic activity was highest when zinc release from the amalgam was the highest. This was from one of the more popular amalgams, Dispersalloy™. Cytotoxic means the substance kills cells. Since amalgam releases mercury, and mercury is bad, and also releases zinc, and zinc is bad, what happens if both mercury and zinc are released at the same time?

Frequently science looks at one variable, but in reality, people do not live in test tubes. We have all kinds of multiple environmental exposures. Why not at least test the combined effects of mercury and zinc, since they both come out of the filling at the same time? After all, a researcher named Chew had tested the long-term dissolution of mercury from a nonmercury-releasing amalgam and found that over 40 micrograms of mercury per cubic centimeter per twenty-four hours was released. This release remained fairly constant during the entire two-year experiment.

The combined results were devastating. The damage to tubulin and creatine kinase from zinc and mercury jointly were far greater than the sum of the two toxicities added together. This meant that far less mercury was required to affect the brain if tiny amounts of zinc were present. Zinc from amalgam enhanced the toxicity of mercury.

After hearing all of this information, I wondered why we don't all have Alzheimer's. Haley had an answer. "Well, that likely depends on whether you have inherited APO-E2, E3, or E4." Oh, yeah, of course, why didn't I think of that? "Genetics is a big factor in whether or not you will develop Alzheimer's," Haley continued. "Genetic research in AD has shown us that the APO-E genes are indicative of susceptibility. We followed this genetic research to see if it correlates with our findings, and it does. Individuals who have inherited APO-E4 genes are far more likely to develop AD than people who inherit the E-2 and E-3 genes. And APO E-2 appears to be more protective than E-3."

"Oh." I said, understanding as much as you do about the matter. Maybe I inherited E-3. "How does this work?" I asked, trying to gain some grasp of what was eliciting so much excitement. APO-E2 has two sulfhydryls and is found in high levels in the cerebrospinal fluid. Therefore, it can bind mercury in the cerebrospinal fluid and protect the brain. APO-E3 has one sulfhydryl, which makes it moderately protective. APO-E4 has lost two sulfhydryls, and does not bind mercury at all, therefore giving even less protection.

"So, in summary if I read you right, your data on the effects of mercury on tubulin and creatine kinase suggest that mercury must be considered as a contributor to the condition called Alzheimer's. Right?"

"Yes," Haley replied, "and this is especially true when mercury is present in combination with other heavy metals such as zinc. Bluntly, the determination of safe body levels of mercury by using animal data, where the animals have not been exposed to other heavy metals, is no longer justifiable. Mercury is far more toxic to individuals when other heavy metals are present. It is my opinion that one of the major questions left to be answered concerning the toxic effects of mercury is: Does the combination of mercury with different heavy metals lead to different clinical observations of toxicity? There is no doubt, in my opinion, that the elevated levels of other metals increases the toxicity of mercury. I also feel that mercury should be in the cross hairs as a target of investigation as a potential strong contributing factor as a cause of Alzheimer's disease."

AIDS and Dental Toxicity

AIDS is another autoimmune disease that can be strongly affected by amalgam fillings. Whether amalgam can be the primary cause of AIDS is not known, but the observations on two patients indicated that amalgam removal clearly improved T lymphocyte counts.

Although this patient sampling is admittedly small, both of these patients (one male and one female) experienced a doubling of their T-cell subsets within a week of amalgam removal. Both patients had already demonstrated the classic suppression of these subset counts typically associated with AIDS.

The increase in the T lymphocyte counts is especially significant in these two patients, since both of them were adamant in declining any of the many other supportive measures we have used to improve immune function. Specifically, no supplementation was initiated, and no dietary suggestions were taken. These two individuals essentially succumbed to family pressure to have their amalgams removed, but they would not compromise their lifestyles any further.

The doubling of these T-subsets counts, then, appeared attributable only to amalgam removal. Even today, there is no drug available that can result in such a stimulation of these cells. Is it possible that removing unnecessary immune challenges (like amalgam) would allow other medications and treatments to have a better effect? This would certainly seem likely. Wondering about the interconnection between immunosuppressive diseases and immunosuppressive materials can lead to some disconcerting conclusions. Experimentally, mercury clearly initiates autoimmune reactions. Perhaps dental amalgam could be a prime player in the etiology of several autoimmune diseases.

Multiple Sclerosis

When you have multiple sclerosis (MS), people are nice to you. As you struggle with your crutches to get through doors, they will hold the door open for you. They help you carry your briefcase up the escalator. For some reason they always tip their head to the side and give a half smile that seems to say, "I'm sorry you have to live that way." Or maybe they are saying, "There but for the grace of God go I," for who knows where MS comes from?

Lots of people know where it comes from. It's just that more people gain by keeping the knowledge under wraps than gain by avoiding the disease. Why do I speak so boldly about MS? Because I've been there. In 1968 I was stricken. Like a lightning bolt. Usually it creeps up on you. I fell in the horse pasture, thinking I had been shot in my leg. The doctor, in fact several, thought I had a broken tendon, and told me that I would be okay in four days.

Four months later, battling doing dentistry with double vision and still on those marvelous, versatile Canadian crutches, I began to doubt I would ever walk again. I did. I skied. I went mountain climbing. I gave up MS. Am I cured? No, just two days ahead of it, and determined to stay that way. If I mess up in diet or supplementation—in forty-eight hours that leg is "gone" again. There is no cure, but there sure is control and improvement available.

In the court trial that took my license (for improving diseases like MS), I was asked if I had been diagnosed by MRI. No, I had to admit. Tricky. That proved I did not have MS. I had MS in 1968 and the MRI was not available commercially until the mid '80s, but legal proof is not always moral proof. Take it or leave it whether or not I had MS. The important thing is that MS and its alleviation got my attention and has resulted in helping over 600 MS patients. We "dentally" treated over 850 MS patients and saw improvement in chemistries and symptoms in about 85% of those folks. From this experience I can tell you, in my opinion, what causes and relieves MS.

Don't forget that word "opinion," for I am entitled to my opinion, even though I have had to fight for it in court. I am definitely opinionated, and those 600 MS patients who improved are one reason for my stubbornness in continuing the battle to stop dentistry from poisoning people with toxic dental materials. You do not have to accept anything I say, but my goal is not to change your mind, just to inform you of what other people are seeing.

How do you "catch" multiple sclerosis? There are two basic requirements. First, you must have a genetic susceptibility, and second, you must have an environmental (meaning originating outside of the body) exposure that triggers the onset of the disease.

For those who are not genetically susceptible, don't worry. You will never get MS. You can have all the mercury, nickel, and root canals you want, and you'll never catch MS. You might get leukemia, diabetes, ALS, or some other autoimmune disease from the environmental exposures to these toxins, but never MS.

In the 1970s we began to notice some characteristics in those people developing MS and started asking questions. First, it was obvious that the vast majority of patients were female. How many? I don't know, but probably over 80%. Dr. Weston Price found an even higher figure in the 1920s, when his studies showed that neurological adverse reactions to dental materials occurred in females over 90% of the time relative to the same autoimmune type of disease in males.

Next we investigated onset. What was going on when you caught the disease? It took a while, but when we saw the connection, it became a repeating process. If a person has an immune challenge, we can label that time as day *one*. If that same person has another immune challenge of equal or greater magnitude twenty-one days later, frequently that was when the genetic weak link broke and disease resulted.

Now let's put that into actual cases. Let's say that you catch a very severe cold (the type that puts you in bed), a case of the flu, have a bout with pneumonia, or get an immunization shot (most are preserved with mercury). Then twenty-one days later you go to the dentist and have an immune challenge from a nickel crown, mercury amalgam, or root canal. You now qualify for MS onset. I mention these initial four challenges because they were the first ones that we observed that related to the twenty-one-day immune cycle.

But what if the challenges are reversed? What if you have the root canal or amalgam, then twenty-one days later you get an immunization shot or catch the flu? No difference. The outcome will be the same. The critical issue is to have the two challenges twenty-one days apart. Now that you are informed, be sure when you go to the dentist that you do not catch a cold twenty-one days later.

Body cycles occur in hundreds of places. We are familiar with eating and sleeping cycles, menstrual cycles, the fact that red blood cells cycle every 120 days, some of the white cells cycle every seven days. Perhaps even biorhythms fall into this category, but there is a whole field of cycles that we never hear about. When I began to look into this area, I soon found several hundred articles that discussed overlapping cycles in relation to everything from the administration of cancer drugs to insulin.

After observing the onset of autoimmune diseases, it became obvious that we were dealing with a 7-14-21-day cycle that even showed up 365 days later. From a practical standpoint, the greatest 7-14-21-day challenge you can receive from a dental office is to have dental appointments scheduled every Tuesday afternoon at 3 o'clock for a month. That is an example, of course, for any seven-day recurring appointment would produce the same effect.

After receiving an immune challenge (day one) you may notice, if you are looking for it, that seven days from then you develop flu-like symptoms. The symptoms only last for an hour or two, then disappear. Your memory usually puts these experiences into the insignificant—"must have been something I ate"—category.

If the subsequent exposure occurs on day fourteen, the symptoms are more severe and last longer. You are actually vulnerable at this time, too, more so than you were on day seven. Should another dental toxic material exposure occur, it is possible for the genetic weak link to break at this time. I have actually seen it happen, but usually one just feels rotten for the day—more so if the exposure was in a mercury-laden dental environment—and the next day you are fine.

It is the twenty-first day that is the most common to notice as the first day you really began noticing the intermittent numbness, the tingling in the hands or feet, the visual disturbances—the first symptoms of multiple sclerosis. It may take months before the symptoms encourage you to seek medical advice. In fact, thirty years ago if someone were coming down with multiple sclerosis it might be years before a diagnosis was forthcoming, and many more years before you were on crutches or in a wheelchair. Now it is more common to see someone go from initial symptoms to wheelchair in three years or less. Why? Do you want my opinion?

I suspect it may be related to the introduction of state-of-the-art high-copper amalgams. Brune showed in the 1980s that the new high-copper (30%) amalgams emitted 50 times more mercury and copper than the conventional amalgams of pre-1980. This figure of 50 times more emission was discovered in a U.S. dental school in the late '70s, but it was elected (with the help of a donation) to keep the information quiet. My opinion is that the combination of the fact that almost all the high-copper amalgams are negatively charged and the fact that 50 times more mercury comes out is a contributing factor to the earlier onset of MS and the more rapid progress of the disease than we had a few decades ago.

In the presence of negative electrical current, mercury is known to be chemically changed into the highly neurotoxic compound methylmercury within less than a second. The trip from the mouth to the sinuses up into the brain requires only a few minutes due to ready transport of methylmercury through tissues. There is no barrier to methylmercury. Plus, it has a high affinity to seek out nerve tissue for a new home.

Once mercury is incorporated into nerve tissue, the contaminated cells look different to the immune system than before the addition of mercury. Immune fighter cells look at the distorted mercury-contaminated cell and identify it as "nonself," or a foreign substance. The job of the immune system is to destroy anything that is not "self," or identified as part of your body. As a result, the "nonself"-appearing normal nerve cell with methylmercury in its structure will be destroyed by the immune system. Your immune system is actually destroying your own cells due to a glitch in identification. The resultant cell destruction is called autoimmune disease. Auto, you, are destroying your "self." And the mercury? It got released from the dead cell so it can contaminate yet another cell. Mercury cannot be "killed."

Treatments usually center on reducing the immune attack, or killing off your own soldiers. Might it be wiser to remove the source of the attack instead of killing our own soldiers? It's a thought. It happens to work more often than not—when the whole protocol is utilized. Just removal of the root canal, the amalgam, or the whatever, in itself rarely produces much improvement on a long-term basis.

Other exposures can contribute to the onset of MS. Some people have been exposed to lead, mercury, and cadmium in homes and businesses built over landfills that were former dump sites for toxic materials years ago. Injuries to the head have been related to MS. Is there a good reason? I think so, yes.

A study was being performed in California on cadaver brains relating the amount of mercury in the brain to the number of fillings. The study was almost finished when the investigators were offered one more brain. This was one from a lady who drove into a telephone pole at about seventy miles per hour. She lived for a bit over an hour, but then died of a severe head injury sustained in the accident. Assays showed that her brain tissue contained over

1,000 times more mercury than any of the other brains the investigators had studied. Did this come as a result of the blow?

As a result of this information, we had a photographer take some infrared pictures that were designed to illustrate mercury coming off amalgam fillings. We put up a black velvet background and touched the filling with a dental drill for about two seconds. The photographs showed the vapor was quite apparent against the black background. It looked similar to smoke curling up from a cigarette.

Later we repeated the photographs and this time used a spoon handle to tap a tooth with an amalgam. Pictures were taken at about one-second intervals and the vapor from simply tapping the tooth rose about an inch each second as shown on the photographs. Could a fall or blow to the head release mercury vapor in sufficient amounts to cause brain damage? What about boxers? The fact remains that we did see a significant number of patients who were involved in auto accidents, falls, or hockey pucks to the head, or some trauma prior to the onset of their MS.

We also suspected that unaddressed or unresolved emotional challenges could affect the immune system in a similar fashion. Nothing definitive here, just acute observations. After all, emotional stress does suppress immune activity. Keep it in mind.

In a few cases, we noted that dentistry could push people "over the edge" without violating the 7-14-21-day immune cycles. In several cases people had amalgams in their mouths and were tolerating them with no apparent problem. Then a broken tooth might result in placement of a gold crown. Gold placed into a mouth with amalgam creates an entirely different electrical "ecosystem." The total electrochemical reactivity among those dental metals can increase as much as tenfold. Several autoimmune diseases have occurred shortly after a crown was placed into a mouth with multiple amalgam fillings. MS is only one of them.

I say multiple amalgams, but actually it only takes one amalgam in some people to create a problem. The total number of different dental materials does affect the time onset of a disease, but not necessarily the outcome. In other words, fifteen amalgams might create a problem in one year, where ten would take two years, but the disease would likely be the same. I have seen a case in which one tiny amalgam appeared to create disease in a very sensitive teenager.

One of the most severe cases I have seen was that of a lady whose problems were initiated by just having her teeth cleaned. Corrosion on the surface of the fillings had greatly reduced the speed of mercury release from her fillings. When the corrosion was removed during the cleaning process and the fillings were polished, the electrical current and resultant mercury escape exceeded her tolerance level.

Does this mean you should never have your teeth cleaned? No. But it does tell you that if you have strange symptoms after having your teeth cleaned, or notice flu-like symptoms seven or fourteen days after that appointment, that you may be in the cross hairs of a future target. To be forewarned can be beneficial. At least you are informed.

Some people catch multiple sclerosis, have their fillings removed, and then go downhill much faster than should be anticipated. As I mentioned before, just taking out the fillings is not a treatment. If the fillings are removed without the protection offered by a rubber dam, suction, and all the other protocol methods, symptoms are apt to get worse.

Fillings are like little tiny batteries. They have an electrical charge. If the fillings with positive electrical charge (as determined by an ammeter that holds the peak amperage) are removed first, leaving negatively charged fillings behind, chemistries and symptoms do not improve much.

If mercury, nickel, and root canals are removed, and replaced with other nonprecious crown materials, or reactive composites (the plastic fillings that can replace many amalgams), then a whole new series of disease events can be initiated.

Many people try to detoxify their systems. This is a necessary procedure, but it must be done carefully. Most of the time detoxification is done too rapidly. Remember, detoxification is retoxification. The body can react to materials as they are coming out of the body.

Where have we seen problems created? In people taking too much calcium, too much magnesium, blue-green algae, spirulina, and the big problem creator, chlorella. Chlorella can be taken prior to amalgam removal with generally no problem. After amalgam removal, it may remove mercury too fast, *or it may contain mercury in the product itself.*

The body responds differently to mercury after amalgam removal than before. This is due to something called a secondary immune response, which is a faster, and more severe, response to exposure to a previously immune-identified toxin.

I could go on and on—which I intend to do in an upcoming booklet just on MS—but it's not fair here to take up much more space. The points to remember here are that mercury can create an autoimmune response. Root canals, as described in their chapter, can generate a toxin that is neurotoxic as well as immunoaltering. Nickel can also create an autoimmune response.

But! That's not all. In the area of toxicology, $1+1+1$ does *not* equal 3. There is a multiplication factor involved in toxicity in which the sum of the toxins is far greater than the total of the toxins. With lead and mercury, for instance, a toxicity rating of 1 for each mercury and lead equals not 2, but 60 when the two are combined. With root canal toxins, nickel, copper, beryllium, mercury, tin, silver, zinc, cobalt, and chromium, in the mouth with just one crowned root canal and one amalgam filling—you can have a plethora of complex toxic reactions simultaneously, made even more complex if you include the cements.

The correction of problems known collectively as multiple sclerosis is complex and detailed, but possible. The important message I bring to you in this book is that much of the problem is avoidable. You don't have to catch MS in the dental office. There are other ways, but at least with dentistry, you have a choice. Don't think so? Yes you do. It is *your* body and you can have it treated or violated in any way you desire. Have compatible dental materials placed in your mouth. Don't allow a bacteria-laden dead stump of a root canal tooth create hardships for your life. Learn what you can about dental procedures and form a team of caring practitioners to aid you before you venture into any extensive dental revision. Above all, you can follow Nancy Reagan's advice when you are offered a toxic material and just say "NO!"

Responsive Symptoms

There are a host of symptoms that respond to dental revision consistently, and we may not have the first clue as to why. Is this any reason that you should not be informed about our observations? I think not. This segment is not meant to be scientific, but just to be added to your wish list of things you would like to see improve. Actually, there are some suggestions as to why some symptoms respond, and they will be mentioned, but some are just happenings. You have a right to know.

Ringing in the Ears

Sure, we are talking about metals in dentistry for the most part, but not the types bells are made from. Why do ears ring? I don't know. In our study of people with ringing in the ears, dental revision helped about 40% of those folks. I remember one patient who was having fillings removed with the rubber dam over her teeth so she could not speak intelligibly. Her eyes were closed and she was very near napping. Suddenly she began speaking in an excited, garbled, wild-eyed gibberish and sat up in the chair. The dentist, fearing a heart attack—for himself as well as the patient—ripped the rubber dam off her teeth and signaled the dental assistant to call 911. When the rubber dam was out, she screamed, "The ringing in my ears just stopped."

You can't hear it, even intimate partners can't hear it, but the victim can—all the time. They reach the point where they ignore it, because like the voice of your conscience, no one else knows what frequency is screaming in their ears. Relief is indescribable—unless you have been there.

Sometimes the ringing stops midstride during the procedures and sometimes it takes a few days. Only one person I can remember had it gradually go away over the period of a month. If you have not "heard" an improvement within a few days, it probably is not going to happen.

Chiropractic Adjustments

More and more people are visiting chiropractors to get their bodies aligned. The problem is that these treatments may turn into a weekly or monthly habit forever. With many of our patients, the adjustments did not seem to "hold." I personally am not sure what the word "hold" means, but I think I have a conceptual idea.

Actually, this was one of first unsuspected benefits to dental revision that was reported to us. People reported that their chiropractic adjustments would hold for months instead of days. Some even reported not having to return for the same old problem anymore. After a while, chiropractors began to call me to discuss the situation. Contrary to my anticipation, they wanted to work together. They were not offended that dental revision had the opportunity to reduce their practice appointments. This offered a nice relationship between health professionals, gave the patient better service, and cost less. It's okay for you to know.

Metallic Taste

Thirty-nine percent of those 1,320 patients reported a metallic taste in their mouths. Where does this come from? The most obvious answer is that there are dissimilar metals in the mouth, and the mouth contains saliva, which is an excellent "electrolyte," or conductor of electricity. With a battery working twenty-four hours a day in your mouth, and metals and metal oxides, sulfides, and sulfates draining out of the fillings onto your tongue, yes, you should have a metallic taste. Copper has the strongest unpleasant taste, but aside from mercury, all the other compounds of metals can produce a disagreeable taste.

Removal of the battery components should eliminate the problem.

But it doesn't always. We have to look to the composition of saliva to gain an idea of why some people don't have the metallic taste until after dental revision. For the most part, the taste goes away with dental revision, but in some cases the body starts dumping metals in the saliva after the fillings are removed. This may continue for several weeks, then gradually decrease until the taste no longer exists.

What metals are in the saliva? The literature abounds with articles monitoring mercury in saliva, so that is a given. But mercury is an odorless, colorless, and tasteless metal. There must be other metals that are being excreted via the saliva. I don't know. This is an area I have never investigated, but would think that copper would be a prime area to look for an answer.

Headaches

Headaches keep several large companies in business. I heard one time how many tons of aspirin are sold daily and it was shocking. Is dentistry related to this industry? Most people feel a drop in intensity of headaches after dental revision. People with migraines will experience a reduction in both number and intensity, such that they do not have to take prescription drugs, and are not debilitated. Over-the-counter drugs will handle the new level. There are some people who will move from migraines to no headaches at all, but this is less than half of the people treated. The usual run-of-the-mill frequent unexplained headaches have a greater tendency to disappear.

I Ferget—(Memory Problems)

Memory loss, especially short-term memory, was present in 58% of our 1,320-person survey. Memory problems can be related to either mercury or to root canals. We have seen it in both cases. Not surprising, it occurs often in dentists and dental personnel. Age is not a factor, for we have seen it in teens as well as seniors. Removal of the offending objects sometimes brings results within days, and there are some folks who just gradually get better over several months. Alzheimer's patients are probably the slowest to recover. Incremental improvements can be seen over a period of several years.

Memory problems are mentioned frequently in texts on mercury in the sections on central nervous system effects. The World Health Organization's 1991 book *Inorganic Mercury* mentions a slowing of the EKG due to mercury exposure as well. Other scientific comments relate to the reduction of cognitive function, but one thing was not expected. There was not a definite correlation between the severity of memory impairment and the amount of exposure. It appears that some people are many times more sensitive than others.

The term "brain fog" was used by Dr. Weston Price as being the comment most of his patients used to describe their condition.

He found this related to people who were reacting to their root canals and thankfully found good recoveries when the offending teeth were removed.

An interesting observation came from the Coors Study. The Adolph Coors Foundation funded many blood chemistries on a series of patients who had testing, amalgam removal, retesting, replacing of the amalgams, then retesting, re-removal, and re-retesting. When we got to the stage of reimplanting the amalgams, the people who were in college had great difficulty in remembering class times, and even one forty-year-old straight-A student flunked a test. All of the participants became argumentative and unpleasant to one degree or another, but certainly noticable by family members within a day or two of the replacement. They had no problem remembering to come in for their final amalgam re-removal appointments, with the hopes of returning to a happier lifestyle.

References for this Chapter

Baasch, E. 1966. Theoretical reflections on the etiology of multiple sclerosis. Is Multiple Sclerosis a Mercury Allergy? *Schweis Arch Neurolochir Psychiat* 98:1.

Brune, D., et al. 1983. Gastrointestinal and in vitro release of copper, cadmium, indium, mercury and zinc from conventional and copper-rich amalgams. *Scandinavian Journal of Dental Research* 91:66-71.

Carandente, F., et al. 1988. Multifrequency rhythms of immunological functions. *Chronobiologia* 15:7-23.

Craelius, W. 1978. Comparative epidemiology of multiple sclerosis and dental caries. *Journal of Epidemiological and Community Health* 32:155-165.

Friberg, L. 1991. Inorganic Mercury. *Environmental Health Criteria* 118. World Health Organization.

Huyltman, P., S. Enestrom. February 1988. Mercury induced anti-nuclear antibodies in mice: Characterization and correlation with renal immune complex depositing. *Clinical and Experimental Immunology* 71 2:269-274.

Ingalls, T. H. 1983. Epidemiology, etiology and prevention of multiple sclerosis: Hypothesis and fact. *American Journal of Forensic Medical Pathology* 4:55-61.

Lawrence, D. A. 1985. Immunotoxocology of heavy metals. *Immunotoxocology and Immunopharmacology*. ed. R. L. Dixon. Raven Press.

Price, W. A. 1923. *Dental Infections, Oral and Systemic*, vol. I. Cleveland: Penton Publishing Co.

Schiele, R. 1988. Statement on uptake of mercury from amalgam. [Institut der Deutschen Zahnarzte]. [Deutcher Arzte-Verlag]. p.123-133.

Schuckmann, F. 1979. Study of preclinical changes in workers exposed to inorganic mercury in chloralkali plants. *International Archives of Occupational Environmental Health* 44:193-200.

Triebig, G., et al 1981. Determinations of motor and sensory nerve conduction velocity in persons occupationally exposed to mercury. *International Archives of Occupational Environmental Health* 48:119-129.

PART III

Sources Of Dental Toxicity

9

Mercury and the "Silver Filling": A Poisonous or Political Issue?

Silver fillings have been called "silver" for their color more than for their composition. Most commercial mixtures are named according to their major component, like wines. If a wine contains a 40%- 30%- 20%- 10% mixture of different grapes, it is likely labeled by the name of the grape that comprises 40% (or the majority) of the wine. With silver fillings containing approximately 50% mercury, 30% copper, 14% each of tin and silver, and 1% zinc, what should the material be called? A "mercury" filling, of course. But we would not knowingly buy a mercury filling because we are aware that it is poisonous. We know it is poisonous, but just how is it poisonous and how much does it take to be poisonous? What does it do to us? That's what this chapter is all about. Science knows what mercury does in the human body. You have the right to know too.

Mercury is poisonous, but did you know that all five of the metals in the silver amalgam filling are poisonous? In addition to that, these metals react with each other and form sixteen more "corrosion products." All of these corrosion products are toxic.

But doesn't mercury stay within the filling? No. The chemical product formed by the "setting" of the five metals is chemically reactive. A mercury vapor meter placed over a filling can detect toxic amounts of mercury vapor within ten seconds.

Fillings release mercury just sitting undisturbed in the mouth, but there are several ways that we can cause our fillings to release increased amounts of mercury. The action of chewing foods increases the vapor escape for an hour or more after we stop eating. The action of chewing gum increases the vapor release due to abrasion as well as by compression of the filling for up to an hour and a half after we stop chewing it. Heat from coffee or other hot beverages increases the vapor release from the fillings.

The electrical charge generated between the various metals within a single filling, or between two different fillings, or between a filling and a crown or braces, releases mercury and corrosion products into the mouth.

How much mercury is released during a day? Is it significant? Articles published in the scientific literature show mercury releases from 20 to as high as 150 micrograms per day depending on the conditions of the study and the type of amalgam. The state-of-the-art high-copper amalgams release 50 times more mercury in a given time than the older "conventional" amalgams. According to Chang at the University of Arkansas, one microgram damages nerve tissue.

The bad thing about mercury release is that it is cumulative. In the fastest elimination mode, if one microgram is absorbed, it will take 70 days to several months to eliminate half of it. Meanwhile, the next day you absorb another microgram, and 69-and-a-half 70ths of the original one microgram are still there. On day three you absorb another microgram, and you still have 69 70ths from the first day, and 69-and-a-half 70ths from the second day, so you can see that even with the fastest elimination, excretion is negligible compared to intake if you have amalgam in your mouth. You will still increase your total body burden of mercury daily.

Not all of the mercury escaping from a filling stays in the vapor form, especially if it is on the surface of a filling registering a negative electrical charge. In the electrical environment on the surface of a filling, mercury vapor is rapidly converted into the highly toxic methylmercury.

Just how many forms of mercury are there in the body, and what do they do? Actually three forms are of primary significance.

The first is mercury vapor. Mercury vapor escapes from the filling, is absorbed through the lungs and intestinal tract, and enters the bloodstream. The primary target for mercury vapor is the brain and central nervous system.

Second is mercury in the ionic form that has two positive charges. Ionic mercury is the *most destructive* form (termed acute and of high magnitude), but its destruction is limited to the area around which it is located. It does not have the ability to move around or through tissues like other forms of mercury. Its damage is usually found in organs like the kidney and the gastrointestinal tract.

The third form is called methylmercury. This is the organic form. On contact with bacteria in the mouth, stomach and intestinal tract, or in the bloodstream, a process called methylation converts both mercury vapor and ionic mercury into deadly methylmercury. The severe toxicity of methylmercury is attributed to its ability to pierce any cell membrane in the body, and cross all barriers, even the placenta and blood-brain barrier. After crossing these barriers, methylmercury is converted back into the highly destructive ionic form, and destroys all cell components in its path. The transportation mechanism into cells is its primary damaging component. Its conversion to ionic form then deposits the "killer" form of mercury in areas it could never penetrate in the ionic form. By this mechanism, methylmercury is credited with creating degeneration and atrophy of the sensory cerebral cortex, paresthesia (numbness and tingling), as well as hearing and visual impairment. In crossing the placenta, it can inhibit brain development of the fetus and create cerebral palsy or psychomotor retardation in the latter stages of development.

Once mercury reaches its destination tissue, it has many ways in which it may express its toxicity. They include the following:

1. Alteration of Cell Membrane Permeability

Each cell is guaranteed its sovereignty by the presence of a cell membrane that selectively lets some chemicals in and keeps others out. When mercury causes interference in the selective mechanism, the cell may absorb the wrong raw materials, and dispense unfinished enzymes or proteins. Cell membranes are rich in sulfhydryl groups, which explains the preference of mercury to bind to membranes. This binding causes cross-linking of proteins within the membrane, which leads to the "leaky membrane" phenomenon.

2. Alteration of Tertiary Structure (Third-Dimensional Form)

Molecules are composed of three-dimensional cloud vapors that react with other molecules because of a mutual fit of their external surfaces. When mercury enters a molecule, it can alter the 3-D form of the molecule such that the key/lock mechanisms no longer fit. This stops the normal chemical reaction that should take place.

3. Alteration of Enzyme Function

Most chemical reactions that the body depends on for daily survival would take hours or weeks to take place in a test tube. Enzymes are proteins that intercede in these necessary reactions by pulling two chemicals closer together such that they react in microseconds instead of days. Mercury can attach to the critical binding areas of enzymes and push the reaction time back to days instead of microseconds.

4. Interference in Nerve Impulses

Nerve impulses travel along nerves. During the trip from the brain to its destination, a nerve impulse does not travel on one continuous nerve. The nerve itself is composed of short segments that intersect at an area called the synapse. Impulses jump the synapse, for there is a space there, between the two nerve segments. The impulse will not jump if mercury is in the gap area. This can result in the end action not happening at all, or happening sporadically due to some impulses getting through, and others not. The resultant sporadic impulses can create tremors and shakes in muscles and altered doses of endocrine hormones to be secreted.

5. Alteration of the Genetic Code

By cleaving our genetic code, called DNA, mercury can cause anything from birth defects in the fetus to altered enzyme formation within brain cells. DNA is a series of purines and pyrimidines linked into a long thread. Two interdependent threads intertwined is the actual form of DNA. Mercury can break one of these threads, leaving the threads attached, but nonfunctional. This is called a single-strand break. It can connect two DNAs together, creating DNA-DNA cross-links, which are the hallmarks of cancer.

6. Inhibition of DNA Repair

Normally when DNA is injured, resulting in a single-strand break, a reductase enzyme repairs the injury immediately. The reductase enzyme is inhibited by the presence of mercury and repair does not take place.

7. Interference with Endocrine Function

Glands that produce hormones are called endocrine glands. Examples of hormones are thyroid, estrogen, testosterone, pituitary, adrenalin, and insulin. Tiny amounts of hormones create major changes in our internal biochemistry, so minute alterations of dosages can severely damage our system. One atom of mercury per molecule can inactivate an entire molecule. Multiple atoms could then be related to "female problems," sterility, lack of energy, and blood sugar fluctuations.

8. Contribution to Autoimmune Disease

Autoimmune disease is a condition in which one's own immune system destroys the cells of his own body. Why does the immune system do this? It is killing your own soldiers. This is a case of mistaken identity. The immune system ignores cells that have your personal genetic code on them. These are called "self" cells. When mercury attaches to a cell, it slightly distorts the shape of the cell (like exchanging a nose for an eye), and the immune system does not recognize it as self. It is called "nonself." Any nonself cell is slated for immediate destruction. Examples of autoimmune diseases are diabetes, arthritis, multiple sclerosis, systemic lupus erythematosus, scleroderma, amyotrophic lateral sclerosis, and AIDS.

9. Digestion and Absorption Alteration

Mercury can kill or alter the digestive bacteria in the intestinal tract, resulting in the formation of abnormal nutrient products. In other actions, it can bind with the intestinal wall absorption pores and electrically reduce absorption of even properly manufactured nutrients.

10. Contribution to the Development of Antibiotic Resistance

Some bacteria alter their form when exposed to mercury. They can do this by adding new genetic material to their DNA. This additive is called a "plasmid." The purpose of developing the plasmid is to allow the bacteria to become resistant to mercury. A side effect of the addition of the plasmid is that many of the bacteria simultaneously become resistant to certain antibiotics. This contributes to the antibiotic resistance problem that generated the need for constant development of new antibiotics. Biochemically, the drug companies are about at the end of the number of combinations of chemicals that can produce new antibiotics.

How much mercury does it take to create destruction? Actually, very little. Let's look at some of the past ten items. How much mercury does it take to disrupt the cell membrane? One part per million (ppm) will alter cell membrane function. Stopping cell growth or reproduction (not addressed) can occur at levels as low as 0.2 ppm. One ppm ionic mercury will substantially reduce the activity of succinic dehydrogenase, ATPase, and alkaline phosphatase in the brain. Glioma cells of the brain are destroyed at 0.2 ppm ionic mercury, and only 0.04 ppm of methylmercury. Even the most resistant parts of the central nervous system are destroyed at 2.5 ppm. Ten ppm ionic mercury will induce cancer-producing DNA-DNA cross-links. This amount can also cause genetic defects. Only 2 ppm of the inorganic form will inhibit the rejoining of single-strand breaks in DNA mentioned earlier. The blood-brain barrier loses its protective selectivity at 1 ppm within hours of administration of either the ionic form or methylmercury.

How many people are actually reactive, sensitive, or allergic to mercury? That depends on who you ask and which question you address.

Sometimes the ADA uses the term "allergic" to describe mercury reactions. That is like being allergic to arsenic or lead. As you can see from the preceding materials, mercury kills cells. Toxicity is not really an allergic reaction, but a pathological disease-producing reaction.

Immunologic Aspects

There are two standard ways of measuring immune activity. We can measure the "viability" of the lymphocytes to get an idea of what concentrations of mercury kill or inactivate our immune system. If lymphocytes are killed, it is a simple matter to stain and count the percentage of dead cells at a given concentration of mercury. Another way to measure immune activity is to measure "immune complexing" in our blood serum. Immune complexing is what happens when our body's immune fighters, called immunoglobulins, or antibodies, come in contact with an invader, called an antigen. In this case mercury is the invader. If blood serum antigen-antibody complexing occurs, the serum is clouded, and the difference in cloudiness can be measured, giving us an idea of the intensity of the reaction.

Using both of these systems, it has been demonstrated that minute amounts of mercury inactivate over 90% of our immune protection system. Our normal immune system has some soldiers to spare, but not that many.

How does the ADA react to this information that over 90% of the population sustains immune reactions to mercury? In June of 1984, the ADA published in *Science Digest* that only 5% of the U.S. population was mercury sensitive (twelve million people) and that was considered insignificant. By the next month, July of 1984, the ADA dropped their figures to 1%, and again claimed that it was insignificant. They compromised at 3% in yet another article, and subsequently said they had only fifty documented cases this century mentioned in dental literature. Of course they excluded all other publications, scientific or trade.

About this same time, the ADA was changing its attitude on what might be called toxic levels of mercury in the urine of their member dentists. In 1983 the Centers for Disease Control (CDC) in Atlanta, Georgia, listed 30 micrograms of mercury per liter of urine as the maximum acceptable level. The word "acceptable" is used because it can't really be called safe. One atom of mercury kills. Zero mercury will never be achieved on this planet, so what is practical? The CDC feels that thirty micrograms is reasonable.

Dr. P. L. Fan of the ADA and Dr. Wilmer Eames, a former dental school professor specializing in amalgam placement procedures, got into what appeared to be a bidding war. Publishing in the ADA newsletter and ADA trade journal, they countered with saying 125 micrograms was safe for dentists, then pushed it up to 150. Next it went to 250, and finally, by the end of 1984, the safe level for mercury in urine was up to 500 micrograms per liter. I (HH) personally asked a CDC official his opinion of this situation. He would not allow his name to be used, but nonetheless offered me a quotation: "It looks to me like an accommodation for sloppy procedures."

Is mercury the only problem?

While taking a master's degree at the University of Colorado in the late '80s, we began investigating blood reactivity to dental materials. It was obvious that mercury created havoc in the immune system, but what about the other components in dental amalgam? My master's thesis was on that topic. All the metals in amalgam were toxic, but not to the same degree. Over the next year, we developed a test for most of the common dental materials including composites, impression materials, crown and orthodontic materials, etc. Varying degrees of toxicity were evident in all dental materials. What's absolutely safe? Only the original tooth. Even examining the materials that were immune compatible most of the time, we would still find that 10% or 20% of people were still highly reactive. There was no pattern. We decided that the "least reactive" materials were best determined on an individual basis and to select them over the moderate or most reactive materials. After all, our immune system is under constant challenge just being on this planet. The air, food, and water are our purest exposures, and even they contain things that cause minor reactions in our immune system.

All dental materials supply some immune challenge, but if we select materials from the least reactive range, we can probably avoid a pathologic response. Now the most reactive materials present a different problem. Many of these, like mercury, copper, zinc, beryllium, nickel, chromium, cobalt, phenol, and others, will forcefully challenge the immune system. When the cumulative challenges from life exposures, together with round-the-clock exposure from dental materials, exceeds your immune defense, disease can result.

Focusing on our 1988 mercury results in the testing of 1,000 people, we found immune reactivity in 89% of those patients. In 1990, the figure on an additional 2,500 people tested from all over the world was 90.2%. Then by 1994 it moved up again, to 92%, and by 1996 it had increased to

94% in testing over 3,000 more people. Why do you suppose there was an upward trend on the same testing? I have a feeling that it is because of the increased use of high-copper amalgam. It releases 50 times more mercury, and has a negative electrical charge on the surface of the filling, which is conducive to the formation of methylmercury. The increase in mercury release plus the addition of methylmercury could explain the overall increase in immune reactivity. At any rate, it is certainly not the 1%, 3%, or 5% suggested by the ADA. You need to be informed of your chances. Mercury's immune reactivity is not to the 100% mark yet. Toxicity, as in killing cells, yes, it is 100%, but in dental materials testing, we are examining only immune reactivity.

What about the safety issues of mercury exposure? Aren't we supposed to be protected by the ADA, the FDA, CIA, someone with three initials? Isn't there a watchdog looking out for us?

Dental associations worldwide generally mimic the American Dental Association policies. To protect the dental industry, both dentists and manufacturers, the associations are forced to defend mercury as totally safe despite their own 1% and 5% figures. As an example, in the March 1971 ADA journal, the editor was asked, "Are amalgam fillings hazardous to the patient?" He replied, "The answer is an unqualified *no*. Study after study shows the patient undergoes no risk . . . the dentist, yes, but the hazard can be reduced to practically zero."

"Study after study"? Despite numerous requests, the ADA has never been able to produce the "study after study" that proves the patient undergoes no risk.

Why? Because there are no such studies.

The British Broadcasting Corporation (BBC) program "Panorama" aired a program in July of 1994 in which interviewer Tom Mangold interviewed Peter Gordon, the scientific adviser of the British Dental Association. From the transcript, Gordon of Britain reflected the ADA views.

> Mangold: "Is amalgam safe?"
> Gordon: "In a word, 'yes'!"
> Mangold: "No doubt about that at all?"
> Gordon: "No doubt about it at all."

The same "Panorama" program interviewed Lars Friberg, M.D., Ph.D., and former head of toxicology for the World Health Organization. As a scientist and specialist in the toxicology of mercury, he had a somewhat different view.

> Mangold: "Dr. Friberg, is there a safe level of mercury?"
> Friberg: "No, there is no safe level of mercury and no one has actually shown that there is a safe level and I would say mercury is a very toxic substance."
> Mangold: "If there is no safe level of mercury, why does the British Dental Association say there is one?"
> Friberg: "I don't know, but I think they're wrong."

If these dental associations think mercury is safe, then why do they insist that dentists use the "No Touch" technique when placing amalgam? Here are their recommendations—and, incidentally, why are they for dentists only?

- Mix amalgam in a closed container.
- Use the "No Touch" technique, whereby placement of amalgam is done with mechanical instruments.
- Work in well-ventilated areas.
- Alert all personnel to the potential hazards of mercury vapor and the necessity of practicing good mercury hygiene practices.

- The dentist must wash his hands immediately after placement into the patient's mouth.
- Store scrap amalgam (left over from placement in your mouth) in a tightly sealed container—preferably under glycerin—and have toxic waste specialists dispose of it.

In response to growing public concern, the ADA produced a pamphlet in 1991 that addressed the critical questions about mercury. Here are some excerpts, with my comments in parentheses.

Statement: Mercury is used in dental amalgams.

Answer: TRUE. When mercury is combined with these metals it becomes an inactive substance. (The sciences of chemistry and physics fail to confirm this statement.)

Statement: Dental amalgams are safe.

Answer: TRUE. Studies have been conducted worldwide for more than 100 years. (Their studies have yet to be disclosed.)

Statement: Amalgam is the most preferred dental restoration.

Answer: TRUE. Other materials have their drawbacks. (According to statements of multiple dental manufacturers in a current California lawsuit over amalgam, the sales of dental mercury in the past ten years have dropped from 220 tons yearly to 34 tons. Many of the manufacturers are offering great discounts to dentists who will buy mercury, but few dentists are taking advantage of this deep discount. The main amalgam market is now third-world countries.)

Statement: Mercury is a naturally occurring element in the environment.

Answer: Mercury is found in food, water, and air. (Uranium, lead, and arsenic are also naturally occurring elements. This is not to be confused with the word "natural" as used in the health food industry. There is an organic form of mercury, too. Want some?)

Statement: Allergic reactions to mercury are very rare.

Answer: TRUE. Fewer than 100 cases have ever been reported. (In the dental trade journals—smart—thousands of reports have been sent to the FDA, but have never been acknowledged by them nor the ADA trade journal.)

To use a favorite quotation from the ADA, but in another context, "There is no scientific evidence that" proves any of their claims.

Scientific evidence of the toxicity of mercury is generously supplied in any of the scientific fields related to biology. This includes immunology, pharmacology, toxicology, endocrinology, genetics, and birth defects, etc. It does not include dentistry.

In another defensive ADA paper, "What '60 Minutes' Didn't Tell You," the ADA claims the "ADA over the years has been supportive of the considerable research that has been done on dental amalgam fillings and welcomes further scientific inquiry."

Experience has shown that the welcome mat to scientific inquiry points out instead of indoors. Many of those dentists who have inquired into mercury toxicity have lost their licenses or been put on probation for challenging the safety of mercury. If a dentist promises to return to placing amalgam and being quiet about the mercury issue, he can just live in fear, but with his license.

I use "he," but there have been several females who have bucked up against the boards in the interest of freedom to help their patients choose; they have been given no better treatment than their male counterparts. I would say worse, in fact, based on the demeaning attitudes of the board members toward women in these cases. One was told that if she thought mercury was dangerous, she must have a psychiatric evaluation before they would even talk to her.

In the state of Colorado, Judge Nancy Connick ruled in 1996 that patients were not allowed to ask a dentist to remove their fillings for toxic reasons. Can you imagine being a Ph.D. in toxicology, asking a dentist to remove your mercury because you know of the toxicity of mercury and choose not to have it in your body, and being eligible for fine and imprisonment?

The rubber meets the road in court. In the "Tolhurst" case in California, the ADA and several dental manufacturers were challenged on the mercury issue. The defense that got the ADA off was "We owe no duty of care to warn of the alleged danger of dental products which the ADA undertakes to research. If such a duty were imposed, it could result in limitless exposure to the ADA for every dental-related injury or illness."

How do you feel about the ADA Seal of Aproval on toothpaste now?

Okay, so the dental industry is scared to death about legal responsibility for continuing to say that mercury is safe, when all the scientific evidence says otherwise . . . it is only logical that they should do everything they can to protect the financial interests of the dentists, the manufacturers, and the insurance industry. I have no problem with that. If everyone who had come down with MS, lupus, arthritis, epilepsy, leukemia, ALS, diabetes, etc., could relate their disease to dental procedures, the ensuing legal battle would be for more money than there is in the universe.

But isn't there someone who is not financially involved? What about the FDA? Aren't they our protectors?

The 1976 U.S. Congress requested that the FDA "classify" dental products including dental silver mercury amalgam fillings. The *Federal Register* recorded another such request in 1980. Multiple requests have been made over the years, yet there is still no classification of dental amalgam.

What is the purpose of FDA classification? Here are some "sound bites" or abstracts from FDA law that may shed some light on the subject of safety. The purpose of FDA classification is "to provide for the safety and effectiveness of medical devices intended for human use (mercury is included here) . . . this law authorizes the Secretary to ban a device which presents a substantial deception or substantial unreasonable risk of illness or injury . . . the Secretary is authorized to restrict the sale or distribution of a device if there cannot otherwise be reasonable assurance of its safety and effectiveness, especially if it is dangerous to health when used as indicated . . . (example) grossly hazardous products such as lead nipple shields which expose nursing infants to possible lead poisoning . . . this procedure is designed to assure that all patients will be informed of newly identified risks associated with the use of a device to which they have been exposed."

In examining the word "risk," the risk need only be a potential one. The risk may be one demonstrated by reported injuries or it may simply be foreseeable.

Just what is this elusive and controversial classification?

Class I materials are those of low health risk. They require no special records or proof of safety. Examples are bedpans and tongue depressors.

Class II materials are those for which reasonable assurance of safety and effectiveness can be achieved through the application of special controls. These controls include performance standards, patient registries, dissemination of guidelines, etc. Examples are orthodontic headgear, and composite plastic dental fillings.

Class III devices are those instruments that are not totally safe, or sufficient studies have not yet been done to allow the FDA to determine potential harm or safety. Class III devices may aid life support more than impede it, as in the heart pacemaker; may be due to public demand, as in the breast implant; or assist people in birth control, as in the intrauterine devices.

The FDA has steadily refused to classify amalgam. They have classified mercury. It is in Class I, of no health risk.

One reason they offer for the Class I registration of mercury is that the health risks are inherent within the device, and that reclassification into Class III where it belongs would not alter the health risks.

This may be a key part of the situation we find ourselves in. Even the governmental agencies have been defending the use of mercury. Perhaps they are protecting each other. Consider for a moment the national consequences if mercury in fillings were reported to be dangerous. The offending parties (dentists, the ADA, and dental manufacturers and distributors in our case), if found guilty, would be submitted to one or more of the following FDA actions:

1. Repair the device so that it does not present the risk. (Mercury can't be removed. If it could, there would

just be powdered metals left, which would be like filling a tooth with sand.)

2. Replace the device with one in conformity. (This could be done by replacing amalgam with composite or gold.)

3. Refund the purchase price of the device. (The ADA says dentistry places 93 million fillings per year. If fillings last ten years, and cost $100 each on the average . . .)

Neale Donald Walsch, in his book *Conversations with God, Book 1,* quotes God as describing how dogmas succeed. Dogmas are organizations such as religions, fraternities, or organizations that guide people's thinking—like the ADA. First, people need to believe they need what is offered. Next, they must lose faith in themselves to be able to do what the organization offers. The organization must have answers that the individual does not. Lastly, the individual must accept the organization's answers without question.

But should you become "enlightened" or exposed to the truth, they must expel and disgrace you with great fanfare, in order to intimidate the membership to continue repeating the herd instinct mantras that are required to maintain status quo. The ADA has certainly achieved these criteria to the letter.

References for this Chapter

American Dental Association. March 1971. Editorial on hazards of amalgam fillings. *Journal of the American Dental Association.*

American Dental Association. June 1984. Percentage of U.S. population believed to be mercury sensitive. *Science Digest.*

American Dental Association. July 1984. Percentage of U.S. population believed to be mercury sensitive. *ADA News.*

Sources of Dental Toxicity

Berglund, A., et al. 1988. Determination of the rate of release of intra-oral mercury vapor from amalgam. *Journal of Dental Research* 67:1235-1242.

Brune, D., et al. 1983. Gastrointestinal and in vitro release of copper, cadmium, indium, mercury and zinc from conventional and copper-rich amalgams. *Scand J Dent Res* 91:66-71.

Chang, L., et al. 1972. Changes in RNA composition of neurons after mercury intoxication. *Fed Proc* 31:665.

Chang, L., et al. 1972. Quantitative cytochemical studies of RNA in experimental mercury poisoning. *Journal of Neuropathology* 31:389-401.

Colorado State Board of Medical Examiners. February 29, 1996. Memorandum from Cathy Lopez, administrative assistant, in the matter of disciplinary proceedings regarding the license to practice dentistry in the state of Colorado of Hal A. Huggins, Case No. DE95-04.

Compeau, G., R. Bartha. 1984. Methylation and demethylation of mercury under controlled redox, pH and salinity conditions. *Applied and Environmental Microbiology* 48 (6):1203-1207.

Federal Register. 1975. Request from Congress that the FDA classify dental products containing dental silver mercury amalgam fillings 40:21847-51.

Federal Register. 1980. Classification of dental devices, development of general provisions 45:85962-86035.

Food and Drug Administration. June 29, 1994. Dental products panel meeting.

Friberg, L., et al. 1986. *Handbook on the Toxicology of Metals*, vol.1. New York:Elsevier Pub.

Gay, D. D., R. D. Cox, et al. May 5, 1979. Chewing releases mercury from fillings. *Lancet* p. 985.

Goncharu, B. A. 1977. Problems relating to occupational hygiene in women in production of mercury. *Gigiena Truda i Professionalnye Zabolevania* vol. 5:17-20.

Huggins, Hal A., D.D.S. 1989. Medical and legal implications of components of dental materials.

Lain, E. S., W. Schriever. 1940. Problems of electrogalvanism in the oral cavity caused by dissimilar dental metals. *Journal of the American Dental Association*, vol. 27.

Ott, K. H. R., F. Loh, A. Kroncke, et al. 1984. Mercury burden due to amalgam fillings. *Deutsche Zahnarztl Z* 39:199-205.

Patterson, J. E., et al. 1985. Mercury in human breath from dental amalgams. *Bull Environ Contam Toxicol* 34:459-468.

Radics, J., et al. 1970. Die kristallinin kompenenten der silberamalgam untersuchungen mit der elektronischen rontgenmikrosorde. *Zahnarzfl Welf* 79: 1031.

Sikorski, R., et al. 1987. Women in dental surgeries: Reproductive hazards in occupational exposure to metallic mercury. *Int. Arch. Occup Envrion Health* 59: 551-557.

Stock, A. 1939. Chronic mercury and amalgam intoxication. *Zahnarztl Rundsch.* 10:371-377 and 403-700.

Tolhurst v. Johnson and Johnson Consumer Products Inc., Englehard Corp., ABE Dental Inc., the American Dental Association, et al. 1992. Case No. 718228, Superior Court, County of Santa Clara, Calif.

U.S. House. 1976. *Medical Device Amendments of 1976.* 94th Cong., 2nd sess. H. Doc. 94-853.

Wranglen, G. 1974. *Corr Sci* 9:331

Wranglen, G., J. Berendson. Circa 1980. Electrochemical aspects of corrosion processes in the oral cavity with special reference to amalgam fillings. *Corrosion and Surface Protection of Metals.* Royal Inst. Technol.

10

A Nickel's Worth of Advice

Nickel is one of the most durable yet most carcinogenic metals on this planet. How did we arrive at the decision to use this combination in children's crowns, braces, adult crowns and bridges, and partial dentures?

When our own teeth succumb to the rigors within the mouth, dentistry is charged with replacing what God made, but with a more durable material; for what God made didn't last. The mouth really is a hostile environment. It is warm, moist, and full of nutrient-laden saliva, decaying teeth, and soggy gums, so it becomes a haven for bacteria. Teeth are also subject to sudden changes of temperature created by extremes such as coffee and ice cream. Mechanical stresses find their way into the mouth in the form of chewing ice and a combination of hard and soft foods. It is attacked chemically by foods that are highly acidic and highly basic with overtones of salinity and sugar.

All these conditions provide corrosive influences for artificial replacements supplied by the dentist. Replacements must be corrosion resistant, strong, thin, and cheap. Nothing satisfies that equation better than the metal nickel. After all, a nickel's worth of nickel will cover a tooth in the form of a crown.

By itself, nickel melts at too high a temperature for normal casting procedures, and does not form accurate margins. When mixed with beryllium, cobalt, and chromium, nickel alloys provide the mechanical properties accepted by dentistry. The nickel content in many dental applications is over 70%.

Another term for nickel compounds is "stainless steel." This fact is not commonly known, for I (HH) have heard many dentists say, "I would not use nickel. It is carcinogenic. I use only stainless steel." Same thing. Where were you in chemistry class?

California's Proposition 65 applies to nickel as well as mercury. This law explicitly states that if you expose someone to an item that can produce cancer or birth defects (reproductive harm, specifically), you must *inform* the recipient before exposing him/her. It does not prohibit you from exposing people, it just says you must inform before you perform.

Let's look at the potential that nickel offers for creating cancer and birth defects, or anything else for that matter. This may help in rendering your informed decision of whether or not you want nickel implanted into your body.

Reports in the *Journal of Dental Research* (1991) demonstrate how nickel dissolves from dental appliances into the saliva. It also reports that if beryllium is present in the alloy (reasonably common occurrence) the corrosion of the alloy is more rapid than in alloys without beryllium.

As far as nickel being carcinogenic (cancer producing) is concerned, that has been published in the scientific literature for over fifty years. Animal studies demonstrating malignancies as a result of exposure to nickel have been shown in multiple strains of rats, mice, guinea pigs, rabbits, and cats.

Most compounds of nickel have carcinogenic properties, just to differing degrees. Alloys producing "soluble nickel ions" create cancer because they can be absorbed across cell membranes readily. This would be the form dental patients would be most apt to encounter. Even greater cancer potential is produced from larger soluble particulates from nickel compounds. These larger compounds must be transported into the cell by a process called phagocytosis, in which the compound is actively "engulfed" by the cell. This is more apt to happen to dental laboratory technicians.

Nickel doesn't just go into the body and produce the same kind of cancer the same place in everyone. It has multiple modes of operation. We should examine several of these so that we can have a better idea of the significance of placing nickel in our mouths.

Here are the primary locations and documented methods of cellular damage caused by nickel.

NICKEL BINDING: Nickel has the ability to bind to oxygen-, nitrogen-, and sulfur-containing biochemicals more tightly than their usual catalysts, magnesium and calcium. Magnesium and calcium are essential in many metabolic activities, and the inactivation of critical enzymes by competitive nickel-binding results in inefficiency of whichever system is attacked. The avenues are numerous and nonpredictable.

GENOTOXICITY: Each day our bodies are confronted with environmental challenges that impact and destroy a small part of our genetic code (DNA) in some cells. These damaged DNAs must be repaired. In addition to that, new cells are being generated at a rate of one million per second. At this speed, even the best accuracy will produce an error in genetic coding every few seconds. This type of genetic alteration can produce cancerous cells, so it is essential that the alterations be corrected immediately. Fortunately, we have an enzyme process that detects and repairs such defects. But, in the presence of nickel, the process can be severely limited or stopped altogether. This can potentially result in the development of a malignancy that without the presence of nickel could have been avoided.

DNA REPLICATION: Replication is the duplication of our genetic code in cells ready to divide. This provides the genetic code for the next generation of cells. Nickel can inhibit the replication process. It can do this by forming DNA-protein complexes in chromatin material, rendering it unable to replicate. One of the worst things it can do in this area is to cause deletions from the DNA during the replication cycle. This ensures that the defect will be passed on to the next generation.

IMMUNOREACTIVITY: Nickel is well documented to adversely react with the immune system. Specifically, nickel is immunosuppressive. The immunoreactivity is particularly evident toward what is called the "natural killer," or NK, cells. These cells are specialized white blood cells from the division called lymphocytes. Their purpose is to locate cancer cells and kill them immediately. They are not required to go through the committee meetings that other white blood cells go through before acting. By inactivating the NK cells, our immediate defense against cancerous cells is eliminated, thus allowing the offending cells to get a better foothold on developing cancer in our bodies. This avenue has been felt to provide the greatest danger of cancer spread of all the problems that nickel creates.

Recent researchers see an entirely different action as being the most significant. Very low, nontoxic amounts of soluble nickel enhance the genotoxicity of *other* carcinogens as revealed by tumorigenicity (the ability to cause tumors) and cell transformation. Exposures to soluble forms of nickel (as come off of dental devices) have a more immediate systemic effect than nickel particles or industrial dust.

Other researchers feel that another reverse-twist action provided by nickel may be of more significance than it has been given to date. There is something called the heterochromatic long arm of the X chromosome that is part of a tumor-suppressor gene. This specific gene helps suppress the development of malignant tumors. Nickel can cause the deletion of that heterochromatic long arm on the chromosome, and we lose some of our natural cancer defense.

An entirely new field of cancer research, the "synergistic interactions between carcinogenic agents," applies to nickel. In this field researchers have found that another metallic cancer inducer, cobalt, enhances the carcinogenic potential of nickel. Cobalt is a frequent companion to nickel as part of the alloy used in dental crowns, braces, and partials.

Copper is another chemical modifier. Copper induces greater carcinogenic activity of nickel than it has by itself. Copper is present in the high-copper amalgams, and is emitted 50 times faster than from the conventional amalgam of a few years ago. Around 90% of the dental gold casting metals contain a substantial amount of copper in order to restore the gold color that is lost in the alloying process with silver, platinum, and palladium.

Back to California's Proposition 65: nickel is listed as a metal that can create "reproductive toxicity." Nickel has been reported to create chromosomal aberrations. What are these? They are disruptive patterns in our genetic code, DNA. Specifically geneticists refer to these disruptions as gaps, breaks, and exchanges. These terms refer to the alterations in the actual chromosomes. Gaps are areas of genetic code that were omitted or removed by nickel. Breaks are DNA strands that have been broken, such that they will produce either none of the proteins that they are supposed to manufacture, or will produce an incomplete protein. Exchanges are segments of DNA that have switched places. This would be like transposing two numbers in your phone number. Would the right connection be completed?

Nickel does even more genetic damage, and this part is difficult because its action is different each time. It directly attacks and alters chromosomes, but not always the same ones. For those of you who are bent toward genetics, the specific chromosomes that have been attacked are numbers 1, 7, 11, 13, 14, 20, and 21. The entire loss of chromosomes 20 and 21 is reasonably common. Another disconcerting part of this action is that these changes are not dose dependent. Extremely low doses (as little as 1 ppm) can cause just as much genetic damage as doses 500% higher. Where mercury would probably kill the cell at these dosages, nickel just makes the cell turn malignant.

DNA damage leading to reproductive toxicity is frequently seen as what are called "cross-links." These are the result of two DNAs fusing or linking, resulting in double the number of chromosomes. By definition, an alteration of chromosomal DNA is a malignancy. Should this occur in a reproductive cell, there will definitely be an increased chance for birth defects or reproductive failure.

Cancer is a serious situation, but not everyone who receives nickel in the dental office is going to get cancer.

There are other things that are not as serious, yet disconcerting, about which you should be informed.

Let's start with small children. At age two, all the baby teeth are in, and I have seen many kids at that age whose teeth are so badly broken down that they have to be crowned. Gold crowns in two-year-olds? No. Chrome crowns. "Chrome crown" is a cutesy name for crowns made of nickel with a splash of chromium and cobalt. These are preformed, hollow tubes shaped like a baby tooth on the top, and can readily be cut down so that they will fit over the broken-down tooth after the decay is removed.

Again, it doesn't happen to everyone, but look in the mouth of a preschooler with "Coke-bottle" glasses. Some of these kids have bi- and trifocals before going to school. Why? Nickel attacks the visual areas of the brain in a similar fashion to that of mercury. Mercury from fillings usually generates nearsightedness, but nickel apparently alters the vision even more. I doubt you will find these observations in the literature, but they are based on hundreds of observations.

Years ago I wrote the book *Why Raise Ugly Kids?*, so I am into observing kids and their specific problems. Many a mother in airports has wondered about me as I walk up to her kid and ask him/her to "open your mouth." They usually respond in proper fashion, and it takes a few microseconds to complete my observation. Chrome crowns stand out like bright headlights. Maybe you have seen them on kid's front teeth. Ugly, yeah, but they are just kids. They don't have feelings when their peers razz them about their appearance. Yes, I am opinionated. Yes, there are better ways, both aesthetically and healthwise.

That kid's immune system has been assaulted with a toxin—a neurotoxin as well as a carcinogen. As kids, the immune system may forgive the insult, but it never forgets. The memory portion of the immune system is called "memory cells." Convenient.

Now let's move up the age ladder a few years and find nickel introduced to the immune system in the form of orthodontic "braces." Now we have added a compounding factor. The kid is in school, bigger physically, under more stress and confinement, and more susceptible to peer pressure. Exposure to nickel at this age, according to physicians I have interviewed, frequently results in a drop in grade-point-average of about 1.5. That means from a B to a C-minus. They may also develop "teenage behavior." Is behavior a factor of age, or a normal reaction to a toxin? Yes, it is both, but one can be avoided, especially if a mercury filling is in the mouth when braces are placed. Check out the literature. Check out the kids blessed with braces. Do I sound irritated? I have talked to those people who were headed for college, then had braces, and were unable to maintain the grades. Now, years later, some of these folks are making the decision to return to college free of toxic teeth and ready to take up where they left off. Sick. It didn't have to happen. They should have been informed.

She had been such a loving little girl, always bright-eyed, and giggling. It had been eleven months since she had giggled. She was a sourpuss with plunging grades. At night she twitched every few seconds. It lasted all night long. Her parents had stayed up to watch. It never stopped.

I have rarely seen a family with such genuine love for each other. I suppose this influenced my decision to see them. I told the father of the potential consequences of my suggested treatment and closed with "if anyone is going to harm her, let it be me." I at least had my eyes open to the problems. He said they would be in the car that night headed for Colorado. Money was no problem. There was none.

The electrical current in the braces made me shudder. I told her father that the current was over a thousand times greater than the brain operated on. I also told him that, in my opinion, if the braces were removed in the wrong sequence in someone with abnormal muscular activity, that something else distressful neurologically could be triggered, and that I had no idea what that might be.

"I guess we'll find out together," he replied.

The braces were removed within my "Bubble operatory," which is surrounded by a Faraday cage. The cage reduces the ambient radiation from radio, TV, CB, and cell phones that can affect people when massive changes are made in the electrical environment within the brain. She did well during the removal procedure. That night she slept without tremors. The next day she began to giggle. Her father (built like a scaled-down King Kong) placed his hands on my shoulders. "You done give me my daughter back," he said. Dry eyes would never have compensated me for my services. I was well paid.

Can braces be made without nickel? Yes. Plastic brackets are available. Gold is coming back, and titanium offers a fine alternative. I contacted one of the major manufacturers of braces and orthodontic wires and told them of the biological hazards. Yes, they were aware. Why don't you change? Why change a good thing (financially)? I was informed that the company already had a policy in place. When they have lost ten cases in courts absolutely proving damage from nickel in their braces, they would change. Their lawyers are ready today.

Let children who had braces move up another decade. A few more life experiences, normal American diet, and we are ready for our first crown. Gold does a very nice job, but nickel is far cheaper. According to the laboratory industry, in the '80s, about 85% of the crowns were made of nickel. This decade is showing a decline due to fear, but we are still faced with over 50% of the crowns being nickel. Dentists are beginning to fear being sued for placing a known carcinogen just because it is cheaper.

Another decade or two of life experiences can result in the loss of a few teeth. How can we replace them? Bridges? Yes, that is an option, or what is called the removable partial denture. Removable partials usually replace more than one tooth. The favorite material is the usual mixture: nickel, beryllium, chromium, and cobalt.

What about those now aging memory cells? Can they still remember? You bet. As a person becomes exposed to nickel, has a few years of recovery, and becomes exposed again, the immune system becomes more sensitive to the new onslaughts. After the second, third, or fourth exposure, the carcinogenic activity is even more apt to be initiated. You need to be informed.

Can anything else be used? Yes, plastic partials are reasonably successful. They do not fit as well as the metal-based ones, but they are satisfactory. Just watch out for the pink plastic holding the artificial teeth in place. The pink color is generally due to mercuric sulfate or cadmium sulfate. Neither one will do you much good. The plastic can be made of clear acrylic, which has no coloring agents in it. Gold makes a terrific partial, but it is heavy and relatively expensive. Titanium is in-between in cost, lightweight, and quite biocompatible.

Let's Hear It!

Ten years ago I was asked to present a meeting in California about the potential hazards of nickel. The request was from the California dental laboratory industry. After an initial conversation about what I would present, the laboratory owners decided it would be best to limit the session to owners only. No technicians would be allowed. A few dentists found out about it and asked to attend. Then the "powers" got wind of the program, and word went out that if dentists were seen at the lecture, they would lose their licenses. With so much threat, intimidation, and possibility of the technicians finding out about what was said, it was decided to cancel the program. What did the powers want kept secret? What you have just learned.

References for this Chapter

Christie, N. T., S. P. Katsifis. 1990. Nickel Carcinogenesis: Biological effects of heavy metals. *Metal Carcinogenesis*, vol. 2. ed. E.C. Foulkes. Boca Raton: CRC Press.

Ciccarelli, R. C., K. E. Wetterhahn. September 1982. Nickel Distribution and DNA lesions induced in rat tissues by the carcinogen nickel carbonate. *Cancer Research* 42:3544-3549.

Cohen, M., D. Latta, T. Coogan, M. Costa. 1990. Mechanisms of metal carcinogenesis: The reactions of metals with nucleic acids. *Biological Effects of Heavy Metals, Volume 2: Metal Carcinogenesis*. Boca Raton: CRC Press.

Costa, M., K. Conway, R. Imbra, W.W. Xin, 1992. Involvement of heterochromatin damage in nickel-induced transformation and resistance. *Nickel and Human Health: Current Perspectives*. pp. 295-303. eds. E. Nieboer, J. O. Nriagu. New York: John Wiley & Sons, Inc.

Robison, et al. 1983. Soluble and insoluble nickel compounds induce DNA repair synthesis in cultured mammalian cells. *Cancer Letters* 17: 273-279.

Wataha, J. C., R. G. Craig, C. T. Hanks. June 1991. The release of elements of dental casting alloys into cell-culture medium. *Journal of Dental Research* 70:1014-1018.

11

Root Canals Revisited

The figures vary, but one thing is for sure. Millions of people have root canals done each year. Estimates for 1996 run from twenty-six million to thirty-five million, yet ask the recipients to describe a root canal, and few can tell more than the basics. It hurt like the devil and cost a lot.

Why does a person even need a root canal? Bacterial infection is the primary reason, followed by trauma. From the practical standpoint, frequently pain is the motivating factor that leads one to the dentist.

Bacteria infiltrating through the dentin tubules under decay can set up housekeeping in the pulp chamber. The pulp chamber is an ideal location for a home, for it is warm, has a constant supply of high quality nutrients, and a waste removal system. If they want privacy, they can slither into the dentin tubules and start communes in accordance with the oxygen supply present. Since there are varying degrees of oxygen deprivation, and each level of oxygen stimulates the bacteria to "mutate" into a slightly different bacterium, a whole plethora of critters can develop from the inoculation of just one bacterium. Over 150 different bacterial strains have been identified at the apex or within the pulp chamber of dead or dying teeth. All but five are classified as anaerobic, or those that thrive in the absence of oxygen.

These bacteria produce waste products known as toxins. The toxins can either be picked up by the drainage system at the apex of the tooth, or flow down the dentin tubules into the periodontal ligament. At the ligament (the interphase between tooth and bone) they can slip into the fluids around the tooth and flow into the bloodstream. They may also be forced up the ligament space into the mouth when the host person bites down or chews. No matter which direction the toxins go, they will be introduced to the innermost portions of the host's body. Some toxins have an attraction for a specific tissue, so may lodge there. Should the bacteria follow the same paths, many of them have a selective predisposition to choose a specific tissue as well.

So, what is involved with a root canal procedure? First, an opening must be made into the pulp chamber. This is usually accomplished with a dental drill cutting through the enamel and dentin into the pulp chamber. Then little tiny files are used to remove the contents of the chamber, be they live, dead, or dying pieces of nerves and blood vessels. Next, the canal is flushed with various chemicals that are designed to kill bacteria. Finally the canal is filled with one of several materials including zinc oxide, calcium oxide and the most popular, gutta percha—a wax material. Since the tooth no longer has a blood and nutrient supply, it will become brittle and subject to fracture, so a crown is usually placed over the completed root canal tooth.

Is it always that simple? No, there may be many interference factors that dictate the outcome of the mechanical success of a root canal. Let's take a few pages to discuss these problems.

Uninformed Consent

1. Finding all the canals can be a problem. Sometimes a single root has more than one canal. Front teeth are supposed to have one, but may have an additional one splitting off of the main canal about one-third of the way up from the apex. These are usually parallel to the primary canal, and will not show up on the X-ray. Multirooted teeth, such as some bicuspids and most molars, have two or three roots. Each root has a primary canal, and may have a second one as well. Lower molars frequently have two canals in one root that sort of blend into each other forming what is called a ribbon canal.

2. Curved canals present a problem, for the files used to cut out the infected dentin are straight. Sometimes a file will penetrate the tooth at the curve, and cut its way out of the tooth missing the curve entirely.

3. Toward the bottom 10 millimeters of the tooth, accessory canals may exit the tooth. There can be a few to several dozen, and they do not show up on X-rays.

4. Removing the dead tissue and bacteria from each of the canals presents the problem of not being able to see whether all the contents are removed or not. It's a dark tiny hole down a long skinny root, and bacteria and debris are smaller.

5. Knowing when to stop at the apex is another trick. X-ray films are shadows, and show an approximation of how long the root is, but they don't tell detail about the end of the root. Sometimes the apex has a dimple in it, and the actual end of the canal is indented relative to where it appears on the X-ray. Filling the canal to the X-ray end would actually overfill the canal. Overfilling is a condition most often apt to create infection, thus the presence of unwanted bacteria.

6. "Sterilizing" the canal is a term that used to be applied to chemically treating the inside of the pulp

chamber. There will often be bacteria in the canal no matter how well you file it. To kill the bacteria, caustic solutions are flushed into them. Many studies on thousands of teeth have scientifically demonstrated the presence of bacteria in 80% to 90% of the canals after they have been "sterilized." Where do they hide?

Dentin tubules within the root of the tooth can harbor millions of bacteria. These tubules extend from the pulp chamber to the outer bounds of the tooth called the cementum. The periodontal ligament and the apex of the tooth still contain bacteria from the original infection. It is impossible to sterilize the tubules, the ligament, or the apex, so the terms "clean" or "disinfect" are gradually replacing the word sterilize.

7. Filling the canals perfectly often defies some the laws of physics. Since 93% of the canals in the U.S. are filled with gutta percha, let us focus on that material. The purpose of filling the canal is to seal the canal from access by bacteria. Several basic principles must be ignored to pronounce the canal sealed. First, the wax is mixed with chloroform to make it soft. The chloroform evaporates, creating 6.6% space that used to be occupied by the chloroform. Punching the gutta percha into the canal creates an elastic rebound just like punching bread dough. Removing the condensing instrument from the canal allows the gutta percha to pull away from the walls of the pulp chamber. Then the final blow, the metal instruments used to condense the gutta percha are heated in order to soften the wax. What happens when heated wax cools? It shrinks—up to 30% the first week after placement. Will that produce a space wide enough for a half-micron- sized bacteria to walk through the apex and up the root looking for a vacant dentin tubule to rent?

If bacteria are the problem creating failure of root canals, why not just load up on antibiotics and kill them all? Or can't the white blood cells of the immune system kill off the bacteria? After all, that's what they are hired for isn't it?

Both the white blood cells and antibiotics face the same problem with root canals. Access. No way can the relatively huge white blood cells get into a dentin tubule. Antibiotics can't get in there, either. And the periodontal ligament? Access is difficult if possible at all. The apex? That should be accessible. It would be, except that in cleaning the canal, frequently debris from filing the canal spills out the end of the root forming a good home for bacteria while providing a barrier for entrance into the canal. Some of the bacteria seem to favor aiding failure of the root canal. Bacteroides is a prime example. Bacteroides species have a form of self-defense. They block the chemical receptors on the white blood cells (polymorphonuclears, PMNs, in particular) so that the cells cannot phagocytize the bacteria. Phagocytosis, or engulfing the bacteria, is the primary way in which white cells destroy bacteria. Other anaerobes, bacteria that live in the absence of oxygen, can also inhibit phagocytosis, thus helping to sustain the inflammatory process.

But are bacteria really the problem? In a sense, no. The bacterial products are the real problem. No white blood cell or antibiotic can destroy the chemicals that are produced by the bacteria around the root canal or infected tooth. These chemicals have been shown in research at the University of Kentucky to kill the most important enzymes in our bodies at *lower* concentrations than the most toxic of organic poisons known. It is impossible to conceive the potential danger these chemicals create. Diseases can be stimulated when these chemicals are present at very little more than the molecular level of concentration. Even one half part per billion can destroy the most resistant enzymes. Inactivating these essential enzymes can lead to many hormonal, neurological, autoimmune, and emotional diseases. They are detailed elsewhere.

What happens when the body realizes that it cannot kill the toxic ingredients proliferating around root canal teeth? In a healthy person, the immune system will attack. It will form pus, soreness, tenderness, and pain—all the things to tell us dead teeth do not belong there. The dentist, anxious to protect his investment in the root canal will usually prescribe broad-spectrum antibiotics in an effort to calm the situation. Antibiotics will eventually halt the immune activity around the root canal tooth, and the pain will subside. The doctor and the patient are now lulled into the satisfaction that the root canal is successful, but the health-wise body undergoes further protection activities. If it cannot loosen up the tooth and exfoliate it, build a wall around it and set up a quarantine, a dense layer of calcium is laid down around the root, giving the X-ray appearance of healed bone. Now the bacteria cannot invade the body, nor can the white cells invade the tooth, so it should be a standoff. What about the chemicals? What about the nutrients? Even though cells cannot cross the calcium barrier, nutrients can get through to nourish the isolated bacteria—and, most important of all—the toxins can flow into the body unimpeded to set up diseases at the tissues of their choice.

Just how strong that calcium layer is can be detected by the dentist who tries to remove the tooth. The brittle tooth usually comes out in multiple smelly pieces after a long battle. The calcium layer, called condensing osteitis, must be removed with a dental burr.

The treatment involved in removing a root canal tooth is complex and covered in books detailing the procedure.

Coverage with intravenous vitamin C to protect against the transient bacteremia that occurs during surgery is very important, yet difficult to find. Dentists are not generally trained in IV procedures. That may change soon. A very short duration antibiotic therapy targeted for the specific anaerobes during that transient bacteremia is also a good idea. Meridian pulses monitored by acupuncturists and acupressurists are found to be "scrambled" after the surgery. One hour of treatment by one of these therapists is invaluable. Ice packs should be administered within minutes after the surgery. If it were possible for the patient to stay in the chair undisturbed for a while after the surgery, it would be advantageous. If all the auxiliary procedures can be accomplished, very little, if any, pain medication is required. If the auxiliary procedures are not available, then fairly strong pain medication must be applied.

Even though the presentation of scientifically proven infected teeth, their toxins, and potential damage have been documented, there is a great deal of resistance from the dental profession to admitting to the potential of root canal teeth being a primary source of "incurable" diseases today. The legal profession and liability insurance carriers are obviously not anxious to confront these problems. While they are arguing about who will be forced to pay, go to jail, and admit wrongdoing, those of you who are more interested in your own health may want to seek treatment in ridding your bodies of the most insidious poison of all times. It will still be years before this information is general knowledge, but you have been informed, and may consent to your own options.

References for this Chapter

Asikainen, S., S. Alaluusua. December 1993. Bacteriology of dental infections. *European Heart Journal* vol. 14.

Debelian G. J., et al. 1994. Systemic diseases caused by oral microorganisms. *Endod Dent Traumatol* 10:57-65.

Gill,Y., et al. August 1990. Orofacial odontogenic infections: Review of microbiology and current treatment. *Oral Surgery, Oral Medicine, Oral Pathology* p. 155-158.

Kolmer, F. A. August 1952. Focal infection in relation to health and disease. *Journal of the American Dental Association* 45:139-159.

Mayo, Charles H. 1913. The relation of local foci of infection to general systemic condition, constitutional diseases secondary to local infections. *Dental Review* 228:281-297.

Price, W.A. 1923. *Dental Infections, Oral and Systemic,* vol. 1. Cleveland: Penton Publishing Co.

12

The Cavitation

What It Is and Why It Forms

A cavitation refers to a toxin-containing hole in the jawbone at the site of a previously extracted tooth. It appears that this hole develops because of incomplete healing after routine extraction. This incomplete healing is promoted by a number of factors, including the following:

Failure to completely remove the periodontal ligament lining the tooth socket.

Physically large surgical excavations, such as with impacted wisdom teeth, where the resulting holes can be expected to be larger than usual and more new bone is required to fill the holes in.

Failure to clean out thoroughly the infected adjacent bone (and infected periodontal ligaments) seen in the extraction of root canals and abscessed teeth.

Failure to remove condensing osteitis, the reactive bone formation that attempts to wall off infection, usually involving the periodontal ligament as well.

Poor systemic healing support from a compromised immune system.

Poor nutrition.

Failure to allow the formation of a complete blood clot at the excavation site, or too early a dislodgment of that clot after extraction; also bleeding disorders.

Smoking.

Antibiotic therapy.

Chronic osteoporosis of the jawbone.

Systemic and adjacent toxicity (from other dental toxicity and other sources).

Preexisting periodontal (gum) disease, in addition to any other factor that would also promote periodontal disease.

One of the primary factors in cavitation formation seems to be that the initial extraction does not include the removal of the periodontal ligament from the socket after the tooth is removed. Unfortunately, this absence of socket cleaning is the way nearly all extractions have been done in the past and continue to be done today. We have published statistical data indicating that this cavitation formation after tooth extraction is the rule and not the exception.

A cavitation can be expected to form routinely when this socket lining separating the tooth from the bone is not removed. One purpose of this ligament is to give a certain amount of natural "spring" or shock absorption to the tooth. Without it, chewing would be much like riding on your rims rather than your tires. When the periodontal ligament is not removed from the socket after the extraction, the surrounding bone receives no notification that the tooth is gone. The remaining presence of the ligament gives the biological message to the surrounding jawbone that all is well, and no new bone growth is needed. Bone cells are not going to start new growth and then migrate through a barrier naturally designed to limit such growth.

The jawbone determines that if the ligament is still there, the tooth must be there as well. However, the periodontal ligament does not extend to the upper edge of the extraction site, approaching the oral cavity. Because of this absence of ligament at the top, new bone growth activity will not be inhibited, and a characteristic, thin cap of bone will eventually extend over the extraction hole. We have also occasionally observed larger cavitations to have only a cap of gingiva, or gum tissue, over them. Even the thin overlying cap of bone does not form in these cases.

This mechanism of cavitation formation also helps to account for the wide variety of sizes and shapes that cavitations assume. Even in the routine dental extraction, portions of the periodontal ligament will sometimes remain more strongly attached to the tooth than the bone and be removed along with the tooth. When partially removed in this fashion, the spotty absence of the ligament will permit equally spotty ingrowth of bone, resulting in the wide variety of cavitation shapes and sizes. Even when the large wisdom teeth are removed surgically from impacted sites with extensive excavation, cavitations are nearly always present. It would appear that when the excavated hole is large enough, cavitation formation can be anticipated even if most or all of the periodontal ligament is removed, since so much more new bone growth is needed to completely fill the hole.

The other factors mentioned above can also significantly promote the formation of a cavitation after the extraction, depending on the particular patient. Condensing osteitis, the bone-hard calcification seen in the sockets of longstanding chronic infection, must be completely removed to give the opportunity for complete healing. Solid, noninfected bone must be reached to allow the normal regeneration of bone.

When infection remains throughout the socket and adjacent bone, with or without condensing osteitis, healing will rarely ever gain the upper hand. Yet the ligament is still not routinely cleaned out even under these circumstances. This inattention stems from the fact that infection is still not realized to be routinely present after the root canal or abscessed tooth is extracted, even when the outline of condensing osteitis can still be seen on X-ray after extraction. If the immune system is already compromised for other reasons, healing will also be inhibited. Poor nutrition promotes poor healing and further suppression of the immune system.

The formation of a blood clot in the healing process does not get the recognition it deserves. Blood clot formation, with its gradual retraction over time as the surrounding tissue heals in, is nature's way of promoting proper healing throughout the body, not just in the mouth. When a nicely formed blood clot fills the socket, healing gets a good start. But when it is dislodged early, or adjacent periodontal disease or smoking causes too rapid a retraction, a dry socket is the result, and cavitation formation can then be anticipated.

Antibiotics to treat the early release of bacteria into the bloodstream after an extraction may have a place in some patients, but a continued course of antibiotics after a thorough cleaning of the socket consistently seems to impair good healing. This negative effect on the healing of the socket should always be balanced by the clinician against the other perceived needs for the antibiotics.

Preexisting diseases, such as osteoporosis with poor bone structure in the jawbone before the extraction, can clearly promote the formation of cavitations. Bleeding disorders, which would directly impair the formation of the important blood clot, can also be promoting factors.

Periodontal disease, which is associated with poorer general health, can also serve to more easily infect the freshly extracted sites and bathe them in the toxins produced by the anaerobic bacteria trapped in the diseased gums. Finally, the presence of local and bodywide toxins will also impair the healing process anywhere in the body. The presence of toxins such as heavy metals will chronically disrupt the calcium/phosphorus balance in the body, promoting the continuous mobilization of calcium from the bone, into the tissues, and out into the urine. Any healing bone needs more bioavailable calcium, not its removal.

Cavitation Frequency

In an article we published in the winter 1996 issue of the *Journal of Advancement in Medicine,* the incidence of cavitation occurrence after routine dental extractions was first pointed out. After routinely drilling at all sites of extraction of the larger teeth in our clinic patients, it rapidly became apparent that cavitations were an *extremely* common finding. It only remained to sit down and review the charts of over 100 clinic patients to see precisely how common it was.

The wisdom teeth, or third molars, were the most commonly extracted teeth in the patients reviewed. Cavitations were found at these sites 88% of the time (313 out of 354 extraction sites explored). The second molars had a 70% incidence of cavitation and the first molars an incidence of 82%. For all molars, the incidence was 85% (441 out of 517 sites explored). As the sites explored were from the extraction of teeth that were smaller, with fewer total root cusps, the incidence of cavitations found declined. The overall rate of cavitations at nonmolar sites was 55% (95 out of 174 extraction sites).

As impressive as these numbers may be for a condition that is still largely unknown to most of dentistry, it should be emphasized that the true incidence of cavitation formation is still probably underestimated by the above numbers. The procedure to clean a cavitation utilizes a blind approach. This lack of guidance can miss smaller and unusually located cavitations. Even a larger cavitation could be missed by the wrong angle of attack, or by failing to explore the one cusp site that had cavitated. Cavitations will also interconnect and form channels in the jawbone. An explored channel might be counted as only one cavitation when it actually developed from more than one unhealed extraction site. Finally, many smaller cavitations will never be found because the operator may not opt to explore a smaller area between the teeth on either side of the old extraction site. Methodology is now being developed that is giving the dentist a computer-generated visualization of the cavitation to be explored. This should also encourage more dentists to perform this procedure, since much less faith that a cavitation is present will be needed when a clear picture can be generated.

Such methodology is also important since most dentists seem to convince themselves that if a cavitation cannot be seen on X-ray, it must not be there. However, a cavitation characteristically *cannot* be seen on X-ray. In fact, this difficulty in being seen on X-ray has caused cavitations to be labeled the "invisible osteomyelitis." While some cavitations can be clearly visualized on X-ray, the vast majority of them, even large ones, will be completely missed on a careful examination of the X-rays. We continue to hear from patients who declare that they are cavitation-free because their dentist looked at their X-rays and declared that none were present. Only the cavitation that has formed with some additional calcification around a well-defined border will be visualized on X-ray. Otherwise, the cavitation just represents one more hole in a sea of many smaller holes, which is the nature of the inside of bone. The bottom line is that a normal X-ray appearance should *never* assure you that no cavitation is present at an old extraction site.

Cavitation Toxicity

Although blunt trauma to the jaw could certainly increase the risk of fracture when cavitations are present, the mechanical consequences of cavitations are not the primary concern. It is toxicity that does the damage. The routine extraction that leaves behind the periodontal ligament and inhibits the formation of a good blood clot also routinely allows the ongoing exposure of this empty socket to the bacteria of the mouth until the top heals over. The cavitation officially forms when healing at the top is complete. The healing over on top allows the rapid development of an oxygen-deprived, or anaerobic, state in the hole. Native mouth bacteria produce highly toxic metabolic by-products as a result of the oxygen starvation. This situation is best understood when one looks at the model of toxicity provided by the feared botulism toxin. Botulism results when a strain of bacteria is similarly deprived of an oxygen environment. Bacteria that normally are harmless to man when oxygen is present form a deadly toxin when that oxygen is removed. This results in the rare but dramatic poisoning seen when vacuum-packed food has these bacteria already present when the seal is made. Also, a subsequent killing of the bacteria will not kill the toxins already formed. Antibiotics will not help the individual poisoned with botulism. Only a rapid neutralization of a large toxin dose will save the patient.

In Chapter 11, the toxicity of root canal treated teeth is addressed. The toxicity of the root canal tooth is also directly related to the toxins formed by bacteria trapped in an oxygen-deprived environment. The toxicity of the contents of the cavitation appears to be identical. Experimental studies have consistently shown toxins in both cavitations and root canal treated teeth rapidly kill vital human enzymes at the lowest imaginable concentrations. In fact, some of these toxins show anywhere from 100 to 1000 times the toxicity of botulism toxin on certain enzymes tested! We are not aware of any known toxins having the potency of bacterial toxins seen in cavitations and other places that trap such bacteria in an anaerobic environment. The clinical toxicity of a cavitation is much more variable than the toxicity in well-controlled experiments with human enzymes. The contents of a cavitation have always tested as highly toxic, but some people seem to do very well clinically when their dental toxicity has been removed except for the cavitations. The reason for this variability seems to be how much access the toxicity has to the rest of the body. The root canal tooth, which is almost always highly toxic clinically, is a tooth that is typically still being used in normal chewing. The root canal, while having had much of the nerve and blood supply removed or damaged by the procedure itself, still has its original attachment to the jawbone. The high pressures generated in chewing can be expected to physically push toxins out of the socket where they can eventually be picked up and distributed by the blood circulation. With the cavitation, however, the pressures of chewing are not routinely transmitted in the same fashion, and the toxins tend more to stay put. Further, some cavitations are very small and are located well above the mandibular nerve while other larger cavitations can even extend below the mandibular nerve. Such larger cavitations would allow the toxins more access to the rest of the body by utilizing the mandibular and other nerve channels.

Cavitation toxicity also tends to be cumulative. The more you have, the more toxicity is present. When the referral center was active, we consistently observed that the sickest patients, usually the wheelchair-bound neurological patients, had the least teeth. Patients who have few or no teeth will usually have long channels of cavitation in their jawbones. In the September 1996 issue of the *Journal of Dental Research,* this observation correlating greater illness with fewer teeth was given support. Joshipura, et al., found that among men who reported preexisting periodontal disease, those with ten or fewer teeth were at increased risk of coronary heart disease when compared with men who still had twenty-five or more teeth, after adjustment had been made for the usual risk factors. Parkinson's disease had long been a disease in which dental revision seemed to rarely have a positive effect. But when cavitation cleaning was added to the program, some degree of positive clinical and laboratory response became routine.

Cavitation Recurrence

Cavitation cleaning, even when done as perfectly as technically possible, does not assure that the cavitation will not recur from lack of complete healing. All the factors already mentioned that can initially cause the cavitation can also increase the likelihood of its recurrence. Patients with larger cavitations and poorer immune systems will often show only gradual reductions in cavitation size as the procedure gets periodically repeated. Each cleaning might stimulate a variable amount of good bone healing before the cavitation process again sets in and the local toxicity prevents further healing.

The primary importance of recurrent cavitation formation is in realizing that it can occur, and not infrequently. When the patient demonstrates good clinical and laboratory improvements and then goes downhill several months later, the possibility of recurrent cavitation formation should be considered in the evaluation of the patient. Other factors should be addressed first, since redrilling the jawbone should not be the first thing done every time the patient gets sicker. Operator skill and proper protocol are important factors in whether a cavitation will recur. The suggested technique for performing cavitation surgery is beyond the scope of this book, but is readily available and quite straightforward.

Cavitation Pathology

As shocking as any aspect of the cavitation is what is routinely found under the microscope. Although most readers might not know one cell type from another, the important thing to realize is that the contents of cavitations are always necrotic, dead material. The microscopic picture looks the same as gangrene! Most people know that the only way to treat gangrene is to cut it out or cut it off. The situation is no different with the cavitation, except that some normal tissue must be entered to reach the cavitation, unlike the black-purple gangrenous finger or foot that everyone knows should come off. And everyone also knows that if a gangrenous extremity is not amputated, the rest of the body will sicken and die. This is also due to a high concentration of anaerobic bacterial toxins. However, when something is out of sight, it tends to be out of mind. Cavitations are rarely apparent; knowing they are there is the first step in getting them treated. Remember that this common condition is really the same as a focal pocket of gangrene in the jawbone.

Laboratory Findings

The effect of cavitations on the laboratory findings is really no different from any other type of toxicity that can target any part of the body. In the Coors Study discussed elsewhere, the spillage of porphyrins in the urine was noted to consistently decrease when the amalgams were removed. We have noted a similar response in urinary porphyrin spillage after cavitation treatment. Other laboratory tests will react depending on how much access the toxicity has to the rest of the body. When someone with cavitations feels well and has a normal laboratory profile, it is likely that most of the toxins are staying in place. But if it is elected not to clean out the cavitations, their presence should never be forgotten if the patient has a subsequent decline in health. Cavitations can progress over time, with more and more adjacent jawbone dying. Cavitations can be relatively stable in size, but they don't have to remain so.

Toxin Neutralization

The approach to minimizing the impact of the toxicity of cavitations is much the same as dealing with all toxins, regardless of source. But when the source of the toxin is identified, as with the cavitation, it should be directly addressed and cleaned whenever possible. Proper nutrition, through proper diet digested as well as possible, is always crucial. All the mineral supplementation appropriate elsewhere is also appropriate in treating the toxicity of cavitations. Vitamin C, in doses of 10 to 15 grams daily, helps most people. If you have any kidney disease and don't like to drink water, lower doses would be in order. Intravenous vitamin C in doses of up to 50 grams over several hours is also highly effective in acutely relieving the negative effects of a large dose of toxicity.

Dental Implants

While perhaps deserving a separate chapter, dental implants are addressed here because they are intimately involved in the toxicity of cavitations. A dental implant involves the direct insertion of a metal anchor into the jawbone, on which a prosthetic tooth is later attached. Any foreign substance, however biocompatible it may be, can be expected to initiate some degree of autoimmune reaction when placed into the body. The dental implant is screwed or planted directly into the jawbone. Removing dental implants was also part of the total dental revision protocol at the referral center.

It was only after we completely realized the toxicity of cavitations that we appreciated perhaps the greatest source of toxicity in implants. The routine approach in implant surgery is to wait a few months after dental extraction, when cavitations are forming, and then to place the implant post directly through this site into the jawbone. Sometimes a full cap of bone has already formed, and the cavitation is completely mature in its toxicity when the implant is inserted. Perhaps the toxicity of implants could be greatly minimized if performed in fully healed bone that had been properly cleaned, but we are not aware of this having been done. In any event, an implant that also implants bacteria and bacterial toxins directly into the bone cannot be expected to have anything but a negative impact on the patient's health.

Public Health Impact

As nearly everyone has had one or more teeth extracted in their life, especially wisdom teeth, the full impact of cavitation toxicity on the public health is enormous. Even young people who have never had a filling, root canal, or crown will often have had their wisdom teeth removed. The toxicity of cavitations can exert its influence over many decades of a person's life. When that person finally gets a chronic or terminal disease, no thought is ever given to the many unnecessary years of toxic stress that the cavitations placed on the immune system. Like the rest of dental toxicity, so many people have it that we have no real knowledge of what life expectancy and quality of health could be without it.

Cavitations also play a prominent role in many people by making other diseases worse. They will make it more difficult for a compromised immune system to ever completely recover. The immune system characteristically tolerates all stresses fairly well until it collapses relatively suddenly. It will compensate as long as possible, then very suddenly its defenses will no longer be effective. As a background toxic factor in many people, cavitations can still serve more to suppress an immune system already collapsed than as a major factor causing the collapse. Just as a boxer can take a jab without falling, the same jab continuously applied after falling will very effectively prevent the boxer from ever getting up again. This is why much of the toxicity from cavitations is so inapparent. It might not be the cause of an illness, but it can easily be the factor that prevents recovery from it. Cavitation toxicity can also be the primary source of toxicity in some people. The lack of awareness of this common condition will remain the main obstacle in getting it routinely treated. Looking for cavitations and cleaning them out should be routinely performed to optimize the strength of any patient's immune system.

Reference for this Chapter

Joshipura, K., et al. 1996. Poor oral health and coronary heart disease. *Journal of Dental Research* 75(9):1631-1636.

Levy, T. and H. Huggins. Winter 1996. Routine dental extractions routinely produce cavitations. *Journal of Advancement in Medicine* 9(4):235-249.

13

Focal Infection

Definition

The term "focal infection" is defined as a localized or generalized infection caused by the spread of bacteria or their toxic products from a distant focus, or site, of infection. Bacteria trapped in specific locations can cause symptoms and diseases far removed from those sites. While focal infection encompasses a range of conditions that goes well beyond those found in the mouth, this chapter is being included to demonstrate to the reader that literally hundreds of years of published research support one of the basic concepts presented in this book. This concept is that infective focal dental toxicity, such as is found in root canals, cavitations, and dental implants, should *never* be overlooked as a cause of many significant medical conditions. Dental infections, a subset of focal infection, have been repeatedly shown to be extremely important factors in causing many diseases. Where the cause-and-effect relationship is less clear, dental infections still almost always make any preexisting diseases and symptoms worse.

Protecting the Root Canal

Bacteria and their toxic by-products have long been recognized as causes of diseases by almost all medical and dental schools of thought. So what's the problem? Simply put, the theory of focal infection strongly threatens the financial backbone of many dental practices, the root canal. The toxicity of the root canal is treated in more detail in Chapter 11, but its method of toxicity is classically that of the focal infection defined above. Since much of the theory of focal infection is accepted by all, those parties favoring root canal treatments needed to do something to try to declassify the root canal as a focal infection. Since the facts were not in their favor, solid supporting research was not a possibility. Rather, a campaign of misinformation was used to promote the safety of the root canal. Whether the root canal proponents truly did not (and do not) realize the toxicity of their procedure is a question that cannot be answered here.

The primary approach of this campaign was simply to state that root canals were not infected, praising the ability of dentists to perform the procedure in a sterile fashion. However, Baumgartner, publishing in volume 2 of the 1976 *Journal of Endodontics*, the journal of those dentists primarily involved with doing root canals, stated that the tooth pulps of root canals were found to grow out bacteria in twenty out of thirty cases. This is a 67% rate of infection for a procedure that aims to be sterile.

Grossman, who is recognized as the founder of the modern field of endodontics, fought hard against calling root canals infected just because bacteria were there. Conflicting with the definition in *Dorland's Medical Dictionary*, Grossman stated that the presence of bacteria alone could not be considered an infection. He claimed that inflammation must be present as well. In fact, other researchers pointed out that inflammation worked to keep bacteria from spreading. This meant that the presence of bacteria in a tooth that *normally should be sterile* would have less difficulty in reaching other parts of the body when inflammation was absent. This also meant that root canals were even more likely to spread bacteria and toxicity throughout the body, since the natural barrier of inflammation was not often substantially present to inhibit that spread. However, many dentists did not want to consider giving up root canals, so they were more than happy to just accept the statement of their leader, not bothering to critically analyze the matter for themselves.

Ironically, Grossman even acknowledged dramatic clinical improvements when root canals were extracted. He simply wrote them off as isolated and insignificant. In one of his articles in the November 1960 edition of *The Dental Clinics of North America*, he stated: "Unfortunately, incidences in which spontaneous remissions occur soon after the removal of a pulpless tooth . . . have led some frustrated practitioners to rely on the focal infection theory as a crutch to offer an explanation for their findings." The term "pulpless tooth" is another name for a root canal. What Grossman either failed to realize or admit to himself was that even spontaneous remissions *must* have reasons for occurring. When a totally unresponsive disease "magically" goes away after something is done, scientific curiosity should be at an all-time high. Sadly, however, when a disease responds in a seemingly incredible fashion shortly after a nontraditional treatment, scientific curiosity appears to be typically nonexistent, perhaps for fear that an unsettling or disruptive conclusion might be reached.

Another perhaps even more unsettling approach to focal infection and the toxicity of root canals comes directly from the American Association of Endodontists. In the fall/winter 1994 issue of *Endodontics*, it is stated that the members of this association are "concerned that misinformed individuals are returning to the research of Price, Rosenow and others—research conducted during the first few decades of this century—and attempting to resurrect the focal infection theory based on these outdated studies." This very disturbing statement implies that good research has a shelf life, eventually becoming useless merely because it gets older. Few physicists would discount any of Einstein's work simply because time continues to pass. Sir Isaac Newton's original observations on the law of gravity still apply today. Yet such statements not only go unchallenged, they continue to get repeated often enough until they get a life of their own. When a statement is made over and over, especially by professionally trained people who are just given respect by virtue of their training, the statement is eventually accepted by many as uncontested fact.

Historical Notes

Focal infection goes back a long way. Even Hippocrates noted correlations between oral infection and remote symptoms. Multiple researchers have associated the removal of sites of dental infection with the improvement of acute and chronic arthritic syndromes. A decayed tooth, when advanced, can also eventually expose the tooth pulp to infection and clinically have the effect of a root canal.

In 1909, Sir William Osler, one of the esteemed founding fathers of modern medicine, credited another early giant in medicine with making the critical correlation between dental infection and so many diseases. Osler credited to Hunter the realization that the mouth was the primary source for the entrance of infection into the rest of the body. Hunter considered infections of the stomach, intestines, appendix, gall bladder, kidney, and lung lining to be largely derived from the mouth.

One of modern dentistry's respected pioneers, G. V. Black, summarized much of the dental literature from the mid 1800s up to 1915. In this summary, he listed at least twenty-eight conditions of the eye as being caused by dental disease, including cataract, conjunctivitis, corneal inflammation, and glaucoma. Among most doctors and dentists today there is no eye condition that routinely triggers the consideration of dental infection as the cause of the eye problem.

Many researchers have noted that focal dental infections can exist for many years without causing any apparent clinical disease. However, it has also been noted repeatedly that good health can disappear rapidly, implying an abrupt and severe loss of immune system protection. This suddenness of immune collapse, occurring far removed from the dental work, probably gives the greatest support to the endodontists' position of the harmlessness of root canals. Although we have repeatedly seen these immune system collapses, mainstream medical clinicians remain most comfortable with seeing immediate and clear-cut cause-and-effect associations between a procedure, such as a root canal, and a disease process. When the immune system finally caves in months or years later to the daily assault of root canal or other focal dental toxicity, the doctor will almost always look for recent, rather than remote, possible causes. And, of course, the patient does not go back to the dentist when his health later collapses. He goes to the physician. The original dentist performing the procedure will usually never know when the patient gets a new medical problem. It's easy to think that you never do harm when you don't do methodical follow-up. And just looking inside the mouth is not methodical follow-up when considering the overall health of the patient.

Streptococcal bacteria were identified as the bacteria most often found in dental infections by multiple researchers. It was also observed that the body forms only a poor immunization to such bacteria, perhaps explaining why streptococci do so much more damage than many other bacterial strains. Historical examples in the literature of the toxicity of the streptococcus, a common inhabitant of the root canal, include the following:

1. In 1931, Cook transmitted colon lesions into rabbits from the streptococci in root canals extracted from patients with ulcerative colitis. Such a cause of this disease is not even considered today.

2. In 1932, Jones found a positive relationship between experimentally produced dental streptococcal infection and cardiac hypertrophy. Such a cause of this disease is not even considered today.

3. In 1928, Nickel stated a specific streptococcus is the common cause of peptic ulcer. Such a cause of this disease is finally being considered today, but only since 1990.

4. In 1936, Swanson would often culture streptococci from "X-ray negative" (normal appearing) root canal teeth. One streptococcus strain, after being recultured from many animals, remained specifically attracted to the central nervous system. Some root canals affect one area of the body, some another. This supported the research of Dr. Weston Price. Dr. Price succeeded in repeatedly transmitting specific human medical diseases to rabbits. Root canal teeth extracted from patients and

implanted under the skin of rabbits would consistently give the *same* disease to the rabbit, even when the same tooth was sequentially used on many rabbits. Dr. Price's experimental work is massive, yet it continues to be ignored today, as root canal treatments remain too massive an industry to be discarded or properly researched.

The above research is but the tiniest sampling of the research done over the last century. The purpose of this chapter is only to make the reader aware of the enormous amount of research already done in this area. The motivated reader can be rapidly overwhelmed by the volume of this research by putting a term such as "focal infection" in a MEDLINE® search category or in any of the search engines on an Internet Web browser.

Other Sources of Infection

The reader should also be aware that there are many other potential sources of focal toxicity, although the dental sources appear to be the most significant in most people. However, when the patient doesn't show a good clinical response to a total dental revision, there should be increased clinical suspicion that another source of chronic bacterial infection might be causing the patient's illness. Other sources of focal infection include the following:

- The tonsils and tissue tags following tonsillectomy— often infection can be trapped in the surgical scar tissue.
- The prostate and the cervix
- The mastoids and the paranasal sinuses
- The gallbladder
- The appendix

The kidneys

Skin infections, such as boils

The colon. A poor digestive system can harbor unpassed
material for years, trapping bacteria without oxygen
and resulting in toxicity.

Periodontal Disease

We have long observed the increased incidence of degenerative diseases in patients with unhealthy, chronically
infected gums (periodontal disease). When one considers
the toxins that bacteria can produce when deprived of oxygen, as in root canals and cavitations, it should come as no
surprise that bacteria trapped without oxygen in diseased
gum pockets can also cause illness. In 1993, the *British
Medical Journal* published that periodontitis increased
coronary artery disease, the primary cause of heart attacks,
by 25%. In 1996, the *Journal of Periodontology* also published material correlating periodontal disease with heart
disease. The message to take from all of this is that infections in the body can have far more than local effects. Bacterial toxins and the further spread of bacteria can often be
the cause of the seemingly unrelated disease being treated.

Treatments

Focal infections generally will respond to the same
measures that are useful in treating other dental infections. Wherever possible, an infected area should be
cleaned out if pus or broken-down tissue is present. The
prime dental examples of this would be the root canal and
the cavitation. Also, when the site is readily accessible and
identified, small subcutaneous injections of protamine
zinc insulin will greatly aid healing. Any oxygen therapy

that effectively delivers more oxygen to the tissues will be very helpful. Magnetic therapy using the proper pole will be very helpful, but inform yourself here before proceeding. The wrong pole will worsen the situation. Mixed-pole applications can also be expected to have long-term negative effects, even when there is short-term improvement. Proper nutrition is critical, and sometimes colonic therapies can help start the lower intestine back on track. Antibiotic therapy should be minimal and closely monitored, as eradication of one infection can promote the development of a new infection, with an unwanted strain of bacteria colonizing elsewhere in the body. Smoking must stop, as it appears to be a primary cause of periodontal disease, in addition to its many other known negative effects. Supplementation should be taken, guided by laboratory testing and clinical feedback.

Parting Thoughts

Although the main purpose of this book is to make the reader aware of the enormous and wide-ranging effects of dental toxicity, the reader should also be aware that not everyone responds as positively to the same treatment. Most people will show clear positive clinical and laboratory responses to total dental revision and proper detoxification measures afterward. However, this chapter is important in letting the reader know that there do exist many nonoral sources of the toxicity we have associated primarily with the mouth in this book. The reader should also know that these sources of toxicity have been the subject of research for centuries.

References for this Chapter

Baumgartner, J., et al. 1976. Incidence of bacteremias related to endodontic procedures: I. nonsurgical procedures. *Journal of Endodontics* 2:399-402.

Beck, J., R. Garcia, G. Heiss, et al. October 1996. Periodontal disease and cardiovascular disease. *Journal of Periodontology* 67(10 Suppl):1123-37.

Billings, F. September 1913. Chronic focal infection on the teeth and elective localization in the experimental production of ulcerative colitis. *Journal of the American Medical Association*, pp. 819-26.

Black, G. 1915. *Special Dental Pathology*. p. 370.

Cook, T. 1931. Focal infection on the teeth and elective localization in the experimental production of ulcerative colitis. *Journal of the American Dental Association* 18:2290-2301.

DeStefano, F., et al. 1993. Dental disease and risk of coronary heart disease and mortality. *British Medical Journal* 306(6879):688-691.

Dorland's Illustrated Medical Dictionary. pp.837-8. Philadelphia: W. B. Saunders Company.

Grossman, L. November 1960. Focal Infection: Are Oral Foci of Infection Related to Systemic Disease? *Dental Clinics of North America* pp. 749-763.

Hunter, W. 1911. The role of sepsis and antisepsis in medicine and the importance of oral sepsis as its chief cause. *Dental Register* 65:579-611.

Jones, N., and S. Newsom. 1932. Experimentally produced focal infection in relation to cardiac structure. *Archives of Pathology* 13:392-414.

Joshipura, K., et al. 1996. Poor oral health and coronary heart disease. *Journal of Dental Research* 75(9):1631-1636.

Kolmer, J. 1952. Focal infection in relation to health and disease. *Journal of the American Dental Association* 45:139-159.

Nickel, A., A. Hufford. 1928. Elective localization of streptococci isolated from cases of peptic ulcer. *Archives of Internal Medicine* 41:210-230.

Osler, W. 1909. *The Principles and Practice of Medicine.* p. 440. New York: D. Appleton and Company.

Price, W. 1923. *Dental Infections, Oral and Systemic*, vol. 1. Cleveland: Penton Publishing Company.

Price, W. 1923. *Dental Infections and the Degenerative Diseases*, vol. 2. Cleveland: Penton Publishing Company.

Quinoz, D. December 1938. Rheumatism from focal infection. *Journal of the American Medical Association* 111:250.

Rhein, M., et al. October 1926. A prolonged study of the electrolytic treatment of dental focal infection—A preliminary report. *Dental Cosmos.* p. 970.

Rush, B. 1818. Medical inquiries and observations. Reprinted in *Oral Sepsis in Its Relationship to Systemic Disease* by W. Duke: pp. 17-20. St. Louis, 1918: C. V. Mosby.

Swanson, W., L. Van Kirk. 1936. Results of culturing 1800 pulpless teeth. *Journal of Dental Research* 15:315.

14

This Won't Hurt—Till Later

To a child, the phrase "this won't hurt" is immediately translated to "what won't hurt?" Children do well in dental offices as long as they are aware of the proceedings. Adults, on the other hand, sit down in the chair (not without trepidation) and just *open wide*. Where the child questions, the adult just trusts.

Dentists, operating from this position of absolute trust, mix materials from unknown composition boxes and deftly implant them permanently into the teeth of unsuspecting and uninformed patients. Physicians must inform their patients of all possible outcomes of intended procedures before performing them. Dentists today are still not obliged to similarly inform their patients. Doesn't the dental patient deserve the same courtesy, and have the same rights, as the medical patient?

One big difference in the two situations is that the physician usually has greater familiarity with the procedure and its consequences. After all, if a patient gets sick, it's the physician who will be the first to be informed. If the dental patient gets sick, the physician is again the first to know, and the dentist is the last to know, and usually never knows. The dentist routinely implants materials of unknown composition and toxicity potential, merely assuming that they offer no harm to the patient. Neither dentist nor patient typically question what is being placed. So, if damage is done, who bears the responsibility? Who takes the blame?

Most sick patients aren't really concerned with finding someone to blame. They just want to get well. Knowing that the problem could have arisen would have been nice, but it is no longer the focus of concern. However, few patients or dentists yet realize that most of the diseases of unknown origin can actually originate in the dental office. Leukemia, diabetes, arthritis, chronic fatigue, infertility, birth defects, emotional instability, nearsightedness, female problems, breast cancer, multiple sclerosis, and Alzheimer's disease are but a few of these diseases. And if the dental office does not mark the onset of one's disease, it can very reliably make any preexisting disease process worse.

As hard as it is to believe such assertions, rest assured that I (HH) didn't believe what was just said a couple of decades ago, either. Yet, I was a dentist who perpetrated all of these afflictions on my patients. But not anymore. I've changed my ways. I seek only to protect my patients, and anyone else who wants to become *informed*.

These assertions are highly inflammatory and very controversial. Can any of these "wild" statements be proven? This book was written so that you can be the judge. We invite you to be the judge, and we want you to be the judge. With the computer age offering the ability to surf the Net and research subjects on MEDLINE®, no one should go uninformed. And no one's assertions should go unchecked or unchallenged. And no one should just trust that everything will be done correctly.

After reading this book, see if you agree that:

Sources of Dental Toxicity

1. Leukemia is a natural reaction of the immune system to protect against invaders that it cannot destroy. It compensates for this inability to destroy the invaders by increasing the number of immune fighters.

2. Diabetes is probably far more an environmental than a genetic disease. A genetic predisposition can certainly play a role, but toxicity plays a primary role.

3. Arthritis pain can be alleviated without the aid of drug therapy. Toxicity must be minimized, and nutrition must be optimized.

4. Much chronic fatigue can be directly attributed to mercury from fillings occupying the chemical carrying sites that are supposed to be reserved for carrying oxygen. Mercury and other heavy metal interference with thyroid activity can also be a contributing factor.

5. Infertility can be related to mercury's toxic effect on sperm.

6. Many studies directly relate a wide variety of birth defects to mercury exposure at different stages of prenatal development.

7. Emotional instability in either children or adults can find its origin in the mouth. The effects of mercury on the thyroid and pituitary glands, aided by some dietary deficiencies, can lead to irritability and aggressive, antisocial behavior.

8. Dentists, with their huge personal exposure to mercury vapor, commit more suicide than any of their contemporaries. Their dental assistants have a 23% higher rate of reproductive failures. Suicide also continues to be a leading cause of death among teens. When added to the typical high-sugar, low-nutrition diet of our current generation, with the contribution of the highly toxic nickel found in ever-present braces in teen mouths, many of these young people face an uphill struggle just to reach adulthood.

9. Mercury fillings and braces can literally sap the intelligence right out of our kids. Braces and declining academic performance go hand in hand. The young person who excels in spite of these added burdens should be viewed as exceptional, with an exceptionally strong immune system.

10. Nearsightedness can be caused by the placement of mercury fillings. The correlation of first amalgam with first glasses will often be apparent, typically within six months of each other. Astigmatism, felt by many ophthalmologists to be a permanent affliction, can improve upon amalgam removal.

11. Female problems are frequently caused or aggravated by mercury toxicity from amalgams.

12. Breast cancer (and other malignancies) can be caused by dental toxicity. Nickel has been cited in more than 1,000 articles as being the most carcinogenic of all natural metals. Nickel is the primary component of most bridges and braces, and it forms the base for many crowns.

13. Dental toxicity is probably a major cause of multiple sclerosis (MS). However, MS is multifactorial, and addressing dental toxicity is not a sure road to improvement, especially when other significant unidentified sources of toxicity are present. Injury to the immune system can have many causes, but the final outcome is often the same. After total dental revision, 85% of the MS patients we have seen showed improvement both in blood chemistries and physical abilities. The spinal fluid proteins of every MS patient we checked showed unequivocal patterns of normalization directly after the total dental revision was completed. Amalgam fillings went commercial in 1832 in Paris, France, the same year that MS was discovered as a disease.

As impressive as the above list of connections between dental materials and disease may be, it is still an extremely limited list, and numerous other equally impressive connections could be added. I (HH) have been known as the "mercury man" for almost twenty-five years now because of the associations between mercury and disease that I discovered. Perhaps what is more important, I have attempted to educate the professionals and the public on the many more such associations already known in history but remaining unknown in modern dentistry and medicine. But my role is only a part of the story.

Perhaps the time for the truth to emerge is now. There is more, much more, to the story of dental toxicity than just the mercury in your amalgams. We all have a right to a fully informed consent before getting our mouths filled with potential toxins. There are alternatives for just about everything. Whatever final compromise is reached in your care should involve your complete and totally informed participation. Remember that it will never hurt to know more. But it could hurt a whole lot to know less.

References for this Chapter

Sikorsky, R. 1987. *International Arch Occup Environ Health* 59:552-557.

Part IV

Post Dental Revision: The Recovery Process Is Only Beginning

15

Proper Detoxification after Total Dental Revision

Basic Terms

At our clinic, patients underwent what we term a "total dental revision," or TDR. This refers to a complete removal of all identifiable dental toxicity, including the following:

1. Replacement of mercury amalgams with bio-compatible composite fillings.
2. Replacement of crowns with more biocompatible materials.
3. Extraction of root canal treated teeth with removal of all surrounding infected ligament and bone.
4. Similarly complete removal of dental implants.
5. Complete cleaning of all cavitations.

The removal of only the mercury amalgams is not a total revision unless no other dental toxicity is present. The unique reactions of the dentally revised patient to be discussed do *not* pertain to someone who has amalgam removed but leaves root canals unextracted. Understanding and remembering the importance of these differences can be critical to the ultimate recovery of the dentally toxic patient. Violation of the principles of detoxification after dental revision to be discussed in this chapter will keep patients ill, or even make them sicker. Some patients are actually better off with no revision at all when these principles are not understood and followed!

The mechanisms of detoxification outlined here represent our best explanations for what have become consistently recurrent clinical patterns. We do not presume to infer that better explanations cannot exist to explain the findings that we have seen. However, the model we are proposing seems to work well in understanding what provokes clinical worsening after TDR. This same model allows us to take precise steps that can consistently reverse these declines in health.

Detoxification of the accumulated heavy metals and other toxins in the body is an important part of the recovery process in the patient affected by dental toxicity. However, the post-TDR patient rarely needs any help at all in accelerating this process of detoxification. Rather, such patients commonly need to find ways to *slow* their rates of detoxification after their dental work has been completed.

Common Detoxification Misconceptions

One of the first misconceptions about detoxification is that it can be completed in a relatively short, defined period of time. By the time patients are in their forties and fifties, with decades of exposure to a wide variety of toxins, the detoxification process can be expected to take the rest of their lives. It will not be over in two weeks, six months, or even five years. The storage sites in the various tissues and organs would appear to have a huge capacity.

Another common misconception about detoxification seems to be that toxins exert no toxic effect while they are being excreted. Nothing could be further from the truth. Detoxification also involves *re*toxification. The degree of detoxification will vary depending on the route of excretion and the types of supplements or drugs being used to facilitate the detoxification. When a toxin has been released from a storage site, 100% of it will not be excreted. Rather, a varying percentage of the toxicity, depending on the presence of toxin neutralizers and the manner in which the toxin was liberated, will be redeposited in new tissues. The primary toxic effect of the previously stored toxin will then be reexperienced to some degree.

Sweating, for example, appears to be one of the least toxic routes of detoxification, resulting in few new toxic effects. Chemical chelators, however, like DMPS or DMSA, consistently produce pronounced amounts of new toxicity as the toxins are excreted. Even EDTA, a consistently safe chelator in patients who have not had a TDR, will often result in clinical setbacks in those who have had a TDR.

Detoxification can also have negative clinical effects through immune system mechanisms. Secondary immune reactions can result in a substantial and acute clinical decline. Such reactions are not generally a problem early in the detoxification period. However, several months or longer after the TDR has been completed, such reactions can appear. When the patient has been very good in avoiding all forms of ingested mercury, which essentially translates into the complete avoidance of seafood, the immune system will sometimes set up a protective mechanism to insulate the body from new exposures to mercury.

Specifically, when mercury-laden meals are ingested after a long-enough period of abstinence, the body will reject the presence of the new mercury. This can manifest as pronounced gastrointestinal reactions, with vomiting and/or diarrhea. Both of these reactions serve to immediately rid the body of the new mercury. Other patients will ingest the mercury without such digestive reactions, but they can reexperience the return of many of the symptoms that had resolved or eased after the TDR. Such symptom return can vary in duration, but typically will last twenty-four to forty-eight hours. It probably is often the real reason for cases of the "twenty-four-hour flu."

If the immune system has had difficulty in recovering, however, symptoms could last even longer. Many people will not experience this secondary immune response, since they never really give up seafood completely. Infrequent but regular meals of seafood tend to inhibit the development of this response. However, it does not mean that the methylmercury in the seafood is not toxic. It only means that you are not benefiting from one of the body's protective responses. Any mercury ingested will accumulate and be toxic, even if acute clinical toxicity is avoided.

The Variable Physiological Response

The same patient who responded *positively* to a specific intervention before a TDR will often respond *negatively* to the same intervention after a TDR. This seeming paradox of clinical response is typically not appreciated by either the patient or the doctor. Understanding the relation of this clinical response to the degree of dental revision achieved is absolutely critical in determining the safest manners of long-term detoxification. Expressed differently, the patient's physiological ability to effectively detoxify will greatly depend on how large a dose of additional daily toxicity is being confronted. When the mouth has been properly cleaned out, the cessation of that large daily dose of toxicity appears to allow the rejuvenation of the body's ability to start naturally detoxifying. It would appear that the typically toxic mouth has almost a paralytic effect on the natural pathways of detoxification and excretion. The poor ability of the pre-TDR patient to effectively detoxify without specific provocative measures suggests that the enzymatic pathways utilized by the cells of the body to eliminate toxins are either neutralized or strongly inhibited by dental toxicity. However, the observation remains that eliminating the dental toxicity restores the body's ability to naturally detoxify, and usually in a relatively rapid manner.

These toxic effects on the ability to spontaneously detoxify consistently produce clinical observations that seem to defy logic. The same drug, supplement, or other measure that made the patient feel better before the mouth was ever cleaned out will often make the same patient feel worse after the mouth has been cleaned out! And this would appear to be because the body's physiological ability to naturally detoxify has been dramatically improved by the elimination of the large daily dose of dental toxicity. The result is that nearly all post-TDR patients need to have their detoxification rates slowed down rather than sped up. However, one of the main clinical objectives of alternatively oriented practitioners of medicine is to get the toxins out, usually as quickly as possible. And when 95% of such a doctor's practice typically still has dental toxicity, the worsening of the clinical conditions of the dentally revised 5% is likely not to be noticed if the other 95% are getting better. That's a percentage rate of improvement that any doctor would be glad to have for just about any condition. But it still doesn't help the poor 5% who have been working so hard to get well and are still getting worse. Most doctors who strive to detoxify patients in their practices believe that toxins already stored in the tissues are uniformly difficult to mobilize and excrete, and they are just not aware of the detoxification differences in the post-TDR patient population.

Toxin Neutralization

How toxic any toxin will be to the body depends directly on a number of factors that relate to toxin quantity and the efficacy of toxin neutralization. These factors are as follows:

1. Rate of appearance of new toxicity. This factor must take into account both the rate of new toxin exposure from the outside and the rate of release of stored toxicity from the inside. Acute and chronic toxin encounters will have different rate factors.

2. Potency of the new toxicity. Certainly, some toxins will compromise the immune system more effectively than others will.

3. Presence of effective, "outside" neutralizers of toxicity. Probably the best example of such a neutralizer is supplemented vitamin C.

4. Presence of effective, "inside" neutralizers of toxicity. A good example of this is dietary and internally synthesized cholesterol, which has been shown to directly neutralize a wide variety of toxins, especially those from bacteria. The quality of nutrition and the synthetic reserves of the body relate directly to this factor.

5. Strength of the immune system. A strong immune system facilitates the contribution of the other factors. A severely weakened immune system lessens

their effects, requiring a much more prolonged period of recuperation and healing.

In conjunction with the above factors, a few general observations on toxicity should be mentioned. Specifically, one should always remember that all substances are toxic at some dose, and a demonstrated toxic effect does not mean a substance should never be readministered. Even excessive amounts of water swallowed can have potentially fatal consequences (noted particularly in some psychiatric patients obsessed with drinking huge amounts of water). However, no one would ever suggest trying to survive without a regular intake of water. Nothing, then, is good for the body that is not balanced by some degree of toxicity, however minimal. Conversely, some agents are toxic at all doses, offering no potential benefit at any dose (e.g., true poisons such as mercury).

The rate of toxin exposure is probably the most important factor in the clinical status of the patient. Outside toxin exposures are well-known causes of clinical illness. Typical examples include acute and chronic toxicity from all of the known and accepted poisons. A much less appreciated source of toxicity results from the toxicity of the detoxification process. Rapidly released toxins from tissue storage sites will reliably result in some degree of clinical toxicity, even if most of the released toxins are eventually excreted. Knowing that these toxins have come from tissue storage sites can usually be implied by the elimination of new outside sources of toxicity in conjunction with the appearance of typical changes in blood, hair, and urine testing. When a patient has not changed anything in his daily routine, including diet, and clinical decline follows the total dental revision, then an accelerated rate of release of toxins from storage tissues can be strongly implied. And when characteristic changes occur in the hair and blood test results, a too-rapid rate of detoxification can be confirmed.

Whether excessive toxicity comes from the inside or the outside, the toxins will reliably induce certain profiles in the biochemical testing. The tests of greatest value for this purpose include serum levels of calcium and phosphorus, cholesterol, globulin, and white blood cell counts. Heavy metal levels in the hair and urine mercury levels are also important. Nearly all of the blood tests commonly tested in a routine checkup can show telltale shifts, but they are of lesser importance to the ones already listed.

Most of the shifts seen on these tests, upon exposure to toxicity, will take place within the established "normal ranges" of most hospitals and laboratories, and would be regarded as meaningless variations by most doctors who regularly work with such tests. Such ranges have to allow the majority of the dentally toxic population to register as normal upon testing. These ranges of normalcy, then, are substantially wider than the ranges of normal that appear in our patient population after dental revision. We have concluded that the majority of the values falling within such normal ranges are really decidedly abnormal numbers, usually reflective of a substantial chronic toxin exposure.

Greater toxin exposure will often result in the following test changes, although exceptions can often occur for a variety of reasons:

1. Calcium/phosphorus ratios greater than 2.5 to 1, with phosphorus levels less than 3.5 mg%. Chronic infections and inflammation in the body can cause opposite trends.
2. Rising cholesterol levels when the baseline levels were 200 mg% or more. Lower baseline levels have

a more variable response, relating to toxin inhibition of cholesterol synthesis and inhibition of cholesterol absorption from cholesterol-containing foods.

3. Globulin levels greater than 2.4 mg%. Levels greater than 3.0 mg% are even more strongly associated with toxicity. Lower levels with much toxicity present tend to occur when digestion remains substantially impaired, or when a diet with inadequate protein building blocks is chronically ingested.

4. White blood cell levels greater than 6,000. Levels below 4,000 relate to longer-term immuno-suppression, and respond less dramatically as toxicity is removed. Lymphocyte count depression appears to be an even better indicator of chronic immune insult.

5. Increase in urine mercury levels. Typically between 4 and 8 micrograms per liter, the level will usually rise. Although mercury is being measured, this test usually "tracks" the excretion of other toxins simultaneously released with the mercury.

6. Hair levels of heavy metals will usually increase. This test responds much more slowly, but when compared with earlier hair results, it is a reliable way to know that toxic body stores are being mobilized.

Other tests will usually show characteristic shifts, but an adequate treatment of this material is beyond the scope of this book. The above is intended only to demonstrate that relatively well-defined shifts will track the internal release of toxicity.

Further Clinical Considerations

The almost uniform appearance of rapid, spontaneous detoxification after a total dental revision is such a reliable clinical response that the absence of such a response should alert the vigilant clinician to one of two possibilities:

1. The dental revision is not complete.
2. A source of daily toxicity greater than that coming from the dental toxicity exists, and should be identified and eliminated.

An incomplete dental revision, which commonly occurs when amalgams are removed and root canals remain, will not usually promote a subsequent rapid detoxification. In some patients, replacement of amalgam with immunoreactive materials will also prevent the appearance of a spontaneous detoxification. However, most people have three or four cavitations at the sites of old wisdom teeth extractions. Leaving these unaddressed will not usually stand in the way of this rapid detoxification post-TDR. However, when many cavitations are present from multiple extractions, they will often prevent the post-TDR detoxification from proceeding if left unaddressed. The variability of this response relates directly to how much new daily toxin exposure remains in a given patient. If only a little is left, detoxification will usually kick in. But if a lot is left, toxins will continue to be retained more readily than they are eliminated.

Because of the above reasoning, the completion of a TDR without spontaneous detoxification suggests a large, nondental source of toxicity. Common examples would include a farmer exposed to large amounts of pesticides, or individuals living downwind from toxic industrial polluters. Many people have very toxic colons, retaining chronic pockets of anaerobic bacterial toxicity of a type similar to some dental infections. Professional colonic therapy can help some of these individuals to eliminate this large source of toxicity. Always look to an incompleteness of the dental revision, first, however. Amalgam tattoos, dental implants, avital teeth, use of incompatible replacement materials, uncleaned cavitations, or even recurrent cavitations should all be carefully considered and addressed first.

Common Detoxification Accelerators

While it cannot be emphasized strongly enough that *any* supplement, medicine, or intervention can potentially over-accelerate the detoxification of the post-TDR patient, there are a multitude of common offenders regarded by most as always harmless. This list includes the following:

1. Many "nutrient food sources," such as chlorella, spirulina, and blue-green algae are common detoxification accelerators. Chlorella is probably the most consistent accelerator of these three. Agents such as these can have dual mechanisms of detoxification acceleration, with an overstimulation of excreting enzymes by bioavailable minerals, and even the presence of trace amounts of heavy metals, promoting the toxicity of the protective secondary immune reaction.

2. Too much of even the best mineral supplements can also overstimulate the detoxification mechanism. If a little is good and even necessary, more is not necessarily better.

3. Some vitamins can have toxic manifestations. B3 will directly promote toxin release, and B12 can promote the methylation of any inorganic mercury present in the body, increasing the clinical toxicity enormously. Very rarely, even a certain dose of vitamin C can promote toxin excretion at a rate in excess of what it can effectively neutralize, resulting in clinical toxicity. But don't stop the C, just reduce it. We have only seen this phenomenon in one patient.

4. Antioxidants can sometimes have unexpected effects. One patient would consistently get recurrent toxic symptoms whenever he took pycnogenol, an antioxidant usually of clinical benefit.

5. Heavy metal chelators almost always overaccelerate the detoxification of the post-TDR patient. DMSA, DMPS, and EDTA can all do this. DMPS is consistently the greatest offender here. Immune declines and clinical illness can result for weeks and sometimes even months after only one injection of DMPS.

Another situation that occasionally occurs bears mentioning. A person who has undergone a TDR might take a supplement early on after the dental work has been completed, and feel better as a result. While that same supplement will likely continue to be a positive support for that individual patient, a patient will occasionally deteriorate clinically after extended use of that supplement. One explanation for this unusual sequence of events is that an occasional patient requires a longer period of time before enough "cellular healing" can take place to allow the cellular mechanisms to speed up the detoxification. Just remember that something good for a while is not always good indefinitely.

Another peculiar reaction deserves special mention. Too much of perfectly good mineral supplements can sicken the patient as effectively as anything. One patient who accidentally started taking sixteen times as much of a mineral preparation as should have been taken demonstrated a rapidly downhill clinical course. In fact, the detoxification in this patient accelerated so rapidly that the liver enzymes dramatically and rapidly rose, reaching the point that a liver biopsy and workup was being proposed. Fortunately, the dosing error was discovered, and the liver enzymes declined again to normal levels after the supplement was stopped. The same mineral preparation was later restarted at the normal dosage, with positive clinical benefit. The patient made a full and complete recovery.

The above example of what an excessively large dose of a good mineral can do raises another concern. Many people will supplement themselves with a wide variety of supplements. Not only do they risk accelerating detoxification too much by the number of different preparations being taken, they also risk overdosing on many of the same minerals being present in the different preparations. Keep things simple, and always note how you are actually feeling.

Immune System Fragility

Always ask: Are my interventions causing *clinical toxicity?* The immune system *never* benefits from being overstressed or overwhelmed. In fact, every such stress can reliably be expected to diminish the long-term recoverability of the immune system. And if the body is symptomatic, then the immune system is being overtaxed, by definition.

Society today tends to admire the athlete and emulates the athletic lifestyle as being healthy. However, it is important to remember that athletic training is predominantly *muscular* training. If you overwork any skeletal muscle in your body long enough and hard enough, you are eventually rewarded with a larger, stronger muscle. Athletes are encouraged to "tough it out," with the promise that their bodies will become stronger and more durable. However, this athletic mindset will hurt the patient vigorously detoxifying. Toughing it out here will not strengthen any muscles. However, the immune system will respond to excessive daily stress by progressively weakening, allowing the strengthening of any disease processes already present or patiently waiting to appear. Several times patients who have tried to do in a few months what should take years have contracted cancer in their detoxification period. Chronic vigorous detoxification rates will reliably compromise the immune system and should be avoided at all costs. This makes perfectly good sense when you realize that a strong immune system is really the only protector between you and any degenerative disease, of which cancer is only one. For a sicker patient, taxing the immune system after a TDR will only start a progressive, downhill spiral in clinical well-being. Never forget the importance of being kind to your immune system.

The contribution of laboratory testing is especially important in regulating this rate of chronic detoxification. Examining a full array of laboratory testing in conjunction with the clinical status is the only reasonably secure way to assure a patient that any sense of well-being is actually attended by good metabolic health. Of course, if the patient is not well clinically, the laboratory testing is less important. But once clinical health is regained, the fine-tuning of the detoxification process requires laboratory testing. Poor test results in a patient feeling well can still indicate an immune system in jeopardy, and further patient management changes that result in normalization trends on later testing are highly desirable. Only then is the patient's immune recovery being given optimal consideration and support.

The basic considerations of immune recovery, then, are worthy of being specifically itemized. We feel that the following points should always be remembered:

1. Clinical decline, or the worsening of clinical symptoms, is the equivalent of a stressed and compromised immune system. The disease or toxicity is winning, and the immune system is losing.

2. Stressing the immune system *never* strengthens it or helps its recovery. A toxin-free body is not an appropriate goal if the immune system must be avoidably traumatized in the process.

3. The more and longer an immune system is stressed, the less likely any significant recovery will result. Immune system trauma must always be considered a cumulative process.

4. The primary goal of the post-TDR patient is to achieve a rate of chronic detoxification that minimizes, or even eliminates, any clinical and laboratory evidence of retoxification while chronically decreasing the total body load of toxicity.

5. *Detoxification done wrong can be worse than no dental revision at all!* This applies especially to heavy metal dental toxicity. However, we would never advocate retaining infective toxicity, such as root canal treated teeth, regardless of how detoxification proceeds.

We offer a practical approach to selecting new supplements or health programs after a TDR. It is an empirical approach, as it must be, since patients can be so variable in their responses to different interventions.

1. List the most prominent symptoms on a piece of paper. List as many symptoms as possible. Rate the severity of each symptom from one to ten immediately prior to starting the new supplement or regimen.

2. Be sure to write the information down; don't just commit it to memory, since the memory is a common target of toxicity.

3. Add up all the numbers in each rating. This is your "severity index."

4. Start the supplement or program in which you are interested.

5. After two weeks, repeat steps 1, 2, and 3.

6. If your repeat severity index number is higher, stop the new supplement or program. Otherwise, enjoy your newfound beneficial intervention.

7. If you clearly worsen or improve before two weeks, the above procedure should not be necessary to tell you what to do.

Immune System Support

The immune system benefits most dramatically when it is directly assisted in the neutralization of toxicity and the nontoxic elimination of toxicity. Nutrition is of critical importance in this neutralization of toxicity. Good nutrition must be maintained on a daily basis to have the most protective effects. Remember that nutrition means the proper diet properly digested. Either poor diet or poor digestion will undermine this protective effect. The body requires a regular source of cholesterol and a balanced amount and variety of the amino acids to protect against toxicity. Butter, eggs, and meats are good source foods. Cholesterol and properly constructed body proteins will help to neutralize toxicity. Vegetarians face an uphill battle in overcoming toxic disease processes. Vegetarians are much more effective at preserving health than at regaining it.

Supplementation should have the guidance of a hair analysis, so that the mineral levels can be more specifically addressed. Hair analysis is not a precise science, but it definitely offers a better guide to choosing supplements over blind guessing or a fixed routine. Supplementation should also be as bioavailable as possible, mimicking the mineral forms found in foods. Nonbioavailable supplements can not only fail to help the immune system, they can also promote toxicity. Calcium is a great example of this. Your body is not designed to assimilate a ground-up rock (dolomite), but manufacturers persist in offering this common, cheap source of calcium to the public. This is comparable to offering a finely ground-up nail as an iron supplement. Such supplements only accumulate where they are not needed, blocking normal cellular function and promoting nonspecifically chronic degenerative diseases. As a very general rule, look for low-milligram, expensive supplementation over high-milligram, cheap supplements. And find a doctor who will follow you, your hair analysis, and your other chemistries to see if the supplements are doing their job.

Vitamin C is probably the single best supplement to directly neutralize whatever toxicity is present at the time. Along with vitamins A and E, vitamin C has been shown to reduce the carcinogenicity of more than fifty air and water pollutants. Frederick R. Klenner, M.D., published papers on the ability of large doses of vitamin C to neutralize the toxicity of snakebite, tetanus, and multiple viruses.

Oral vitamin C is desirable on a regular basis, but the immune system especially seems to respond to the support of large intravenous doses. Fifty-gram infusions over two to four hours will almost always result in an immediate improvement in clinical well-being. Lesser doses are also beneficial, but irrational fears of "mega-dose" vitamin C should not prevent its optimal usage.

The immune system is also best served by avoiding too much physical exertion. Exercise in moderation is great, but it can easily be overdone, especially in a patient already trying to bolster a chronically weakened immune system. Watching the recovery of our sickest patients taught us that exercise should never be taken beyond the point of very early or mild fatigue. More than that can induce its own clinical decline. The mechanism is unclear, but it could also represent a connection with detoxification acceleration. However, regardless of the mechanism, overexercise can crash the immune system.

Conclusion

The purpose of this chapter is important and simple: Addressing dental toxicity only *begins* when the dental work is completed. Much more can be written on this subject, but such detail is beyond the scope of this book. Just be aware that proper detoxification deserves an equal amount of attention as the proper removal of the toxicity from the mouth.

References for this Chapter

Klenner, F. 1971. Observations on the dose and administration of ascorbic acid when employed beyond the range of a vitamin in human pathology. *Journal of Applied Nutrition* 23:61-88.

Klenner, F. 1948. Virus pneumonia and its treatment with vitamin C. *Southern Medicine & Surgery* 110:36-8.

Klenner, F. 1949. The treatment of poliomyelitis and other virus diseases with vitamin C. *Southern Medicine & Surgery* 111:209-14.

Klenner, F. October 1958. The clinical evaluation and treatment of a deadly syndrome caused by an insidious virus. *Tri-State Medical Journal* 11-5.

Smith, L. 1988. The Clinical Experiences of Frederick R. Klenner, M.D. *Clinical Guide to the Use of Vitamin C*. Portland, OR: Life Sciences Press.

16

Some Observations on Sleep and Dreams

There is a whole series of changes that occur during dental revision procedures. Some of these have substantial support in research, like improvement in function after removal of the toxic materials mercury, nickel, and root canals. Others happen and you need to be informed, even though I (HH) have not the first clue where these changes originate in the brain. For instance the change from dreaming in black and white to dreaming in color. This is not life threatening, but it does indicate that something happened. Good or bad? God only knows, but you deserve to be aware of these potential changes so you don't think you are nuts. It's happened to others.

Autoimmune diseases frequently produce alterations in sleeping patterns. Some of these diseases include multiple sclerosis, Lou Gehrig's disease, Parkinson's, Alzheimer's, arthritis, diabetes, leukemia, and others. In most people, this translates into sleeping more hours; in a small percentage, sleep will be decreased to three hours per night. With extensions of up to nine or ten hours, one credits it to chronic fatigue and doesn't think much about it. When people extend their sleeping time up to eighteen hours or more, they know they have a problem.

There is a good scientific reason for alteration of sleep patterns from both mercury and from root canal toxicity. Both can interfere with the function of acidic fibroblast growth factor (aFGF). This is an enzyme that controls our sleeping and eating cycles. Science is just now discovering that it controls many other biologic functions, but sleep will cover what we are looking for now. Ultra small amounts of the toxins from root canals (down in the parts per billion range) can reduce aFGF by 50% or more. This can definitely affect sleeping patterns.

Let us start with the question: What is the purpose of sleep? In babies and children, growth takes place when they are asleep. As a child is growing it needs greater sleep to accomplish this task, extended sleep is normal. No problem.

In adults, the healing process is active when we sleep. If we have had an injury, we require healing time, thus more sleep. That is biological also. No problem. We also deal with maintenance. During the day we may accumulate toxins and DNA breaks, and waste products from the day's metabolism. All cells have a projected life span, after which they have to be removed and new ones manufactured. Red blood cells are a good example of that action. A red cell lives approximately 120 days, then is recycled. The body manufactures about one million red cells per second. That means that there are approximately one million per second that have to be removed. It takes time to clean out all that material, so we sleep to accomplish that task. No problem with this either.

What is going on with people who sleep ten hours or more? They have more metabolic cleanup to do. Constant bombardment by mercury from fillings and toxins from root canals can take more time than the allotted seven to eight hours. This will be especially true if the person is also consuming caffeine and alcohol from beverages, sugar and chocolate in the diet, and junk food far astray from the ancestral diet.

Another thought to factor in is that toxic metals like those encountered in dental fillings can slow down the energy-producing mechanisms (take porphyrin production, for instance) that are required for cleanup. Heavy metals in particular alter the cell membrane function, which changes the rate at which nutrients are taken in and waste products are eliminated. Accumulations of carbon dioxide within a cell can reduce its efficiency and require more metabolic energy for disposal tasks. The selective choices of what is absorbed or not absorbed can be drastically altered by toxins. Put all of these things together, and the result is inefficiency, which leads to longer times for recovery; thus, the requirement for more sleep.

A small percentage of mercury-toxic patients experience a drop in sleep requirements—serious drops, like down to three to four hours per night. This is not a healthful situation either, for it is pushing the body to perform cleanup tasks at a higher rate of speed than is biologically sound, and it may not be as efficient. Metals can supercharge or overexcite nerves such that a smaller stimulation is required to elicit an overresponse. Ever have a sunburn? Remember how sensitive your skin was if someone patted you on the back or clothing rubbed on the burned area? This is an example of overstimulation to damaged tissues. This condition can also be called insomnia, and blamed on psychological factors. Mercury operates in that arena also, so who knows just which factor is the major problem?

Let's talk about dreams. This is an area in which people keep quiet because they don't want to be thought of as a mental case. With slight encouragement and letting patients know others have experienced the same thing, I have observed a common pattern. Many people have recurring emotional nightmares about their teeth. They are falling out. Sometimes someone is knocking them out, but more often the teeth just fall out by themselves. Sometimes one at a time, but mostly, all the teeth just fall out at once. Now these folks dare not mention these dreams to friends or family, but it's okay to talk with us about it. After dental revision, they do not have these recurring nightmares. Interesting.

On the topic of nightmares, many people report that the frequency of nightmares in general is greatly reduced post dental revision. And here is one that is better yet. Many people report dreaming in black and white prior to dental revision, then they dream in color afterward. The reason behind this is totally unknown to me and I have found nothing in the literature referring to this phenomenon. I once attended a conference along with 200 psychologists on the topic of dream interpretation. They were all authorities in this area. At the question-and-answer session, I described the black-and-white switch to color and asked for an explanation for this phenomenon. I got 200 blank stares, and the panel mumbled something about, "We'll look into that and get back to you." If any readers know why this happens, please let me know. The panel has had five years, so I don't anticipate an answer from them.

Color dreamers report that the dreaming experience is far more pleasing than their black-and-white episodes. They say that their dreams are more relaxing and happy even though they cannot remember much about the context.

At this time, I can only propose: May your dreams come true.

Conclusion

What is the reader to believe after reading this book? Can two authors really know so much that remains unknown to so many others? In fact, a growing number of health care providers like ourselves are aware of many of the issues that we have raised. Alternative, nontraditional forms of health care are increasing in number and availability every day now. However, the support of the status quo should never be underestimated. At least two major movements in the last 150 years against the use of mercury in the mouth were ultimately defeated by the promercury forces.

Throughout the history of science and medicine, those in power have vigorously opposed anyone who does not agree with them. Why this phenomenon exists is not easily explained. One reason is control. Those in control want to remain in control. To acknowledge the validity of the opinions and observations of others is considered a sign of weakness and loss of power. Closely associated with this power is the desire to be given due respect for one's accomplishments. When one discovery can potentially eliminate the significance of the life research of others, the predictable reaction will be hostile rejection, not amazed acceptance. Although the public very much wants to believe that the primary motivation of their health care providers is the welfare of their patients, this is often not the case.

It is not our intent, however, to make blanket statements attacking the integrity of our health care providers. Many, perhaps most, of these professionals simply never become aware of most of the information in this book, so their consciences may be legitimately clear. What is less understandable is the efforts of so many of these people to avoid the opportunities for education. Most dentists who strongly oppose most of the concepts we've discussed have never made their own evaluations. Rather, they accept blanket statements from their governing organizations that "numerous studies show" whatever is being promoted. Dentists, physicians, and all other health care providers have a sacred duty to their patients that cannot be passed along to someone else. To just know that there are strong opposing opinions on a subject such as amalgam and not take some time to read original articles, not opinions on articles, is inexcusable. Patients place a total trust in their doctors. The outcome of an ill-advised decision can mean a deformed baby, unnecessary heart surgery, or years of costly and needless medicine.

Science at all levels should continue to strive to become what it has historically never been: open, objective, and receptive to all new theories based on their scientific merit *alone*. Our greatest scientific advancements have consistently come from the few or the one. Einstein, Galileo, Newton, and Tesla are some good examples. If the majority always ruled, progress would never occur. Even today, getting valid research published in a recognized journal is an imposing challenge when the information does not agree with mainstream thinking or when the importance of prescription drugs is minimized. The true validity of the research remains irrelevant.

The legal system has been a major player in blocking the scientific pioneer. The courts have almost blindly supported the majority scientific view. Critical decisions on scientific opinion have been routinely thrown back by the courts to the traditional scientific organizations for analysis and evaluation, with a uniformly predictable result. The organization will never rule against its own policies or beliefs, yet the structure of the court system has consistently asked the majority if the opposing minority has a valid point. It has been said, and it is probably true, that real scientific advances only occur when an opposing generation dies away, and the new generation grows up using the previously "radical" point of view from the start.

True progress will only begin when intellectual arrogance dies. The primary attribute of the scientific mind is humility, not intellect. Only when intellectual curiosity is stronger than the fear of being wrong or humiliated will science grow rapidly and positively. Many people are suffering needlessly and dying needlessly because of intellectual arrogance. A scientist, and especially a clinician, must always have both the mind and the heart open, or the suffering will continue.

Suggested Resources for Help and Additional Information

Suggested readings:

It's All in Your Head: The Link Between Mercury Amalgams and Illness, Dr. Hal A. Huggins, Avery Publishing Group, Inc., Garden City Park, N.Y., Copyright 1993

Root Canal Cover-Up, George E. Meinig, D.D.S., F.A.C.D., Bion Publishing, Ojai, Calif., Copyright 1996

'New' Trition, Dr. George Meinig, Bion Publishing, Ojai, Calif., Copyright 1987

For further education and assistance:

Peak Energy Performance, Inc. (PEP)
4680 Edison Avenue, Suite A
Colorado Springs, CO 80915
Telephone: 800-331-2303 (office)
           719-548-1600 (office)
Fax: 719-572-8081
E-mail: dentaltox@peakenergy.com
Website: www.peakenergy.com

PEP provides serum biocompatibility testing, as originated by Dr. Huggins, to help guide patients to the least toxic replacement fillings and dental materials. PEP also carries a variety of educational materials and nutritional supplements. Programs are offered to assist the patient in minimizing the difficulties encountered in detoxification after the removal of toxic dental materials.

Write to either author in care of this publisher or

Contact Dr. Huggins at
Telephone: 719-522-0566
Fax: 719-548-8220
E-mail: hahuggins@hugnet.com
Website: www.hugnet.com

Contact Dr. Levy at
Telephone: 719-548-1600
E-mail: televy@medmail.com.

Index

K

misleading assurances concerning, 223–225
removing, 205–206
toxins generated by, 145, 159, 163

S

Seafood, mercury content of, 44, 56–58, 82–83, 243
Secondary immune response, 82
Seizure accompanying completion of dental revision program, 124
"Self" cells, 30, 79
Sensitive people. *See* Chemically sensitive people
Serum biocompatibility testing, 66–69
Serum cholesterol levels, 99
Serum phosphorus, 115
Silver mercury fillings
actual composition of, 169
instability of, 40
Sleep, changes in, 22, 259–262
Smoking, 230
Sperm, mercury's effects on, 41
Spermicide use, 54, 117
Stainless steel crowns, 190
Stem cells, 138
Sterility, 116. *See also* Fertility
Streptococcal infections, 227–228
Suicide, 111–113, 235
Supplements, evaluating, 251–253
Symptomatology, 160–164
low-grade chronic, 20
Systemic Lupus Erythematosus (SLE), 29, 31, 142–144

T

Teenagers, mercury's effects on, 113
Tertiary structure of cells, alteration of, 172
Testes, mercury accumulation in, 41
Testosterone, 115, 117
Thimerosal, 56–57
Thyroid hormone, 107–110
effect on dental decay, 107–108
Thyroiditis, Hashimoto's, 31
Thyroid stimulating hormone (TSH), 109–110
Titanium, 198
Total dental revision (TDR)
defined, 241. *See also* Dental revision program
Toxicity. *See also* Detoxification
of metals, 25, 47, 169–170
neutralizing, 218–219, 246–249
protection against, 102
reproductive, 193–194
Toxin magnification phenomenon, 48
Tubulin, 145–147

U

Unipolar magnetic fields, effect on biological systems, 15
Urination, 114
Urine
mercury in, 249
porphyrins in, 71–72, 75
specific gravity of, 112, 114
Uterus, mercury accumulation in, 115

V

W

X

Z

About the Authors

Hal A. Huggins, D.D.S., M.S.

Of the thirty-six years he has been practicing dentistry, Dr. Hal Huggins has spent thirty years developing a multidisciplinary approach to treating dentally toxic patients. Although he still spends most of his time in his home state of Colorado, he now travels a great deal, helping to develop centers around the world to offer treatment using his approach.

In 1973, he was introduced to the concept of mercury toxicity from silver mercury fillings and soon discovered a multitude of incurable degenerative diseases that seemed to be related to the placement of mercury in fillings. He returned to the University of Colorado for a master's degree with emphasis on immunology and toxicology as the first step on his quest to reverse a health situation that he sees as having worldwide implications.

So far, that quest has taken Dr. Huggins to forty-six states and thirteen foreign countries, where he has lectured a total of 1300 days and given 970 media interviews, all on the topic of dental toxicity. He has treated 2,000 patients for the condition.

This is Dr. Huggins' third book. He is also the author of *Why Raise Ugly Kids?*, published by Arlington House in 1981; and *It's All in Your Head*, by Avery Publishing Group, 1984. He has also written about fifty articles and papers on the subject of dental toxicity.

Thomas E. Levy, M.D., J.D.

Dr. Thomas E. Levy obtained his bachelor of arts degree from the Johns Hopkins University in 1972. He then graduated from the Tulane University School of Medicine in 1976. He is board certified in both Internal Medicine and Cardiology. After completing his postgraduate training at Tulane, he served as an assistant professor of medicine at Tulane Medical School for three years. After being in the private practice of cardiology for about fifteen years, Dr. Levy received his law degree from the University of Denver in 1998.

Dr. Levy has worked with Dr. Hal Huggins for about the last five years on dental toxicity issues. He has also served as the medical technical adviser to the International Tesla Society for the last four years, writing articles in the Society's journal on fluoridation, dental toxicity, AIDS, vaccination, and nutrition.

Hampton Roads Publishing Company

. . . for the evolving human spirit

Hampton Roads Publishing Company
publishes books on a variety of subjects including
metaphysics, health, complementary medicine,
visionary fiction, and other related topics.

For a copy of our latest catalog,
call toll-free, 800-766-8009,
or send your name and address to:

Hampton Roads Publishing Company, Inc.
134 Burgess lane
Charlottesville, VA 22902
e-mail: hrpc@hrpub.com
www.hrpub.com